Stop Losing Sleep Over the Size of Your Butt

5 simple truths to help you fall madly in love with yourself

MISTY TRIPOLI

ISBN: 978-0-5789-6064-0

Contents

Introduction   1

Chapter One:
The Beginning of Bulimia   7

Chapter Two:
Fitness Industry Lies   15

Chapter Three:
The Groove Truths   25

Chapter Four:
No One Cares   33

Chapter Five:
Do it Your Way   41

Chapter Six:
No One Can Do it For You   51

Chapter Seven:
You Must Apply It   59

Chapter Eight:
The Discover Your Groove 30 Day Challenge   67

Chapter Nine:
What Others are Saying   152

Introduction

*"There's no prerequisites to worthiness.
You're born worthy, and I think that's a
message a lot of women need to hear."*
- Viola Davis

Without a doubt this was the lowest point of my life. Years of abusing my body with bulimia had culminated in me waking up on my bathroom floor covered in vomit and blood. Yes, it really was as disgusting as it sounds. And yes, I knew what I was doing to myself was killing me. But knowing this wasn't enough for me to stop. Being tired of hating myself, lying to people I loved, being a fraud to my clients... none of it was enough to stop. I knew I had to change but I had no idea how. I felt totally hopeless and wondered if things would ever get better. Or, was this as good as it gets?

The question, "Is this as good as it gets?" resonated over and over in my mind. The very thought of being back on this floor one year, five years or ten years from now gave me such a feeling of despair that I could hardly bear it. I was just so tired of abusing my body and treating myself with such disdain. If I couldn't figure out a way to get better, I simply didn't want to go on.

Perhaps coming to such a dire realization was the catalyst for what happened next. While lying on this floor, embarrassed, confused, desperate and afraid, I had a profound awakening that would eventually lead to my healing. A voice inside of my head, that got progressively louder, repeated the words... You are Enough! You are Enough! YOU ARE ENOUGH!

The louder this voice grew, the more the anger and frustration that I'd been experiencing about not having a "perfect, flawless" body began to disappear. It was replaced with an assurance that I no longer needed to worry about what I looked like, or what others thought about me. That I didn't have to doubt my self-worth. That I really was enough!

Now, while this might not seem like an incredible, earth-shattering revelation to anyone else, for me it was huge. In this moment of clarity my mind was literally transformed and for the first time that I could remember, I felt at peace with who I was and what I looked like. Plus, I could see a path whereby I was going to be able to appreciate my body for all of the unique and amazing capabilities that I had been blessed with.

A path where I wouldn't have to constantly compare myself with others, to hate myself, or abuse my body.

Armed with this new hope, I began a quest to become truly healthy. Both on the inside and out. While it took some time, and a lot of trial and error, I'm happy to say that the path I discovered has allowed me to completely change my thoughts around food, my expectations about my body, my perspective on exercise, the manner in which I talk to myself, how I interact with others, my relationships, as well as virtually everything else in my life. This has led to an almost unlimited amount of confidence, fulfillment, satisfaction and happiness. Plus, I no longer suffer from bulimia.

Now that I've discovered this path for myself, I've made it my life's mission to share what I've learned with others so that they can discover their own path to vibrant health and happiness, too.

Hi, my name is Misty Tripoli and I've been in the fitness industry for over 30 years. During this time, I've seen it all - and taught it too. The hundreds of different workout routines and programs, the endless array of fad diets and gimmicky products, the rise of the mega-gyms. There's always some new and shiny product when it comes to "helping" people lose weight. However, even though the programs and products continue to change, one thing that hasn't changed is the fitness industry's obsession with a person's outward appearance, and how they correlate this with being healthy. Sadly, this emphasis on appearance isn't allowing people to actually get healthy, and more often than not it leaves them feeling like they're not enough. It certainly did for me.

The truth is, the notion that being skinny or thin means being healthy is just nonsense. When I was suffering from bulimia, I may have looked okay on the outside, but I was anything but healthy on the inside. That's because thin doesn't mean healthy!

After finally coming to this realization for myself I knew there needed to be a fundamental shift in the way I approached health and wellness. It was this desire that led me to develop something totally different than anything out there.

Something that focused just as much attention on getting healthy on the inside, as getting healthy on the outside...

Something that allows you to move your body in a pain-free, gentle manner, yet that still challenges you physically and creatively...

Something that would teach you how to truly love yourself and accept your body. Not at some point in the future, but right now...

Something that would help you cultivate

practices and habits that would allow you to experience the true, vibrant health that you deserve.

I am proud to announce that this journey has culminated in the creation of my health and wellness program - Body Groove. However, it's probably not appropriate to even call Body Groove a program. It's actually more of a philosophy of how to best treat your body to maximize your health and happiness.

While Body Groove incorporates all the normal things that you'd expect in a wellness type "program" - like exercise and healthy eating - it's built on the foundational principle that you are a unique individual with unique, individual needs. So, what works for one person won't necessarily work for you. Your body is different and you should move it in a way that's best for you, not some "cookie-cutter" approach to the masses.

While this might sound obvious, it's remarkable how the fitness industry ignores this. For them, it's all about "follow-the-leader" and do exactly what they do. But this is rarely what is best for your body.

For me, when I stopped following the "experts" and started trusting my own intuition and doing things my own way, that's when everything changed.

That's when bulimia left me...

That's when I effortlessly dropped the extra weight that my body had been carrying for decades...

That's when, for the first time in my life, I started to love who I was and love my body...

That's when I began to experience the real happiness that I had always hoped for and knew that I deserved...

That's when I was able to appreciate the fact that I was enough!

I want you to experience this too. To avoid having to struggle like I did! To avoid feeling like a failure because you couldn't stick with someone else's plan. To love and respect yourself for all of your unique characteristics and abilities. To discover your own, personalized path to vibrant health and happiness!

The only thing I ask is that you begin this journey with an open mind, and with the desire to think and do things a little differently.

So, if that's you, and you're looking for a pathway to true, vibrant health... then I'd love for you to join me. I can promise you that it will change your life. Just like it has for me and for so many thousands of people all around the world.

Join me!

Chapter 1

The Beginning of Bulimia

"I said to my body, softy: 'I want to be your friend'.
It took a long breath, and replied: I have been
waiting my whole life for this."

Nayyirah Waheed

I grew up with women everywhere in my life. Six sisters, my mom, my grandmother, tons of aunts. Just women everywhere. What I didn't realize at the time, but realize now, is that none one of these women - who I love dearly - actually liked their bodies. As a young girl, this had a very profound effect on me.

You see, every time one of these women complained about how they hated their thighs, or they had to lose weight, or compared themselves negatively to someone else, it reinforced a notion that in order to be beautiful I had to be thin. Or, in order to love and appreciate my body, I had to look a certain way.

Without knowing it, the actions of the women in my life were causing me to obsess about my size and to find fault with my body. It's no wonder that growing up I hated the way I looked. I was merely copying the example of everyone I knew and admired.

What about you? How many women do you know who really love their body? My guess is not many. Sadly, this is the case for most women.

Now, here's an even scarier question. How many of you, through your actions and words about your body, are negatively impacting the women and girls you interact with? Perhaps your daughters, your nieces, your friends? Is your example teaching them that the only way they can be happy about their body is if they're thin?

Even if you're doing a good job for those around you, your example is only a fraction of what your loved ones are exposed to. They are bombarded with hundreds and thousands of images every single day on television, in magazines, and on social media that associate beauty, wealth, fame, popularity, and even intelligence, with how you look. It's almost impossible to find anyone or anything that isn't reinforcing the idea that to succeed in life you have to be thin.

For me, this barrage of outside negative influence started when I was about 14. Like many young girls, as I hit puberty my thighs and hips started to grow and this was really upsetting to me. To complicate things, being a teenager in the '80s I was exposed to the likes of MTV and fashion magazines, and I remember looking at these women on TV and in these magazines and recognizing that my body was very different to theirs. This really bothered me.

In fact, I was so angry with my appearance that I used to grab my thighs in total disgust and verbally reprimand myself for being what I considered to be disgusting and fat.

Truth is, I wasn't either!

Like most young girls, and most women, I constantly compared myself to others and the images I was being exposed to all the time. It didn't matter what I actually looked like because in my mind I wasn't good enough. As women that's part of our dysfunction. We're never satisfied! We never think we're enough.

"It's almost impossible to find anyone or anything that isn't reinforcing the idea that to succeed in life you have to be thin."

Here's where my story took a tragic turn. At this delicate age of fourteen years old, I watched a movie about a girl who suffered from bulimia. At the end of the movie this girl actually died. However, as much as I believe the producers of this movie were trying to expose the dangers of eating disorders, that is not what I took from watching it. Instead, I found myself saying, "Oh! That's the secret. I can eat whatever I want because I can just throw it up afterward."

So, at around fourteen years of age I started making myself throw up and thus began my sixteen-year battle with bulimia.

Now, I couldn't actually make myself throw up. Instead of sticking my fingers down my throat I would drink this stuff called Syrup of Ipecac. It's what you give babies to make them throw up if they have been poisoned. I was just so determined to get thin that I was willing to do anything.

My Life as a Fitness Trainer

A couple of years into my battle with bulimia, I developed another obsession. Working out.

At around 16 years old I walked into a gym and watched people teaching a dance type aerobic class and knew that I could do that too. So, I got a job teaching step aerobics. I then ended up going on to teach everything else too. Every kind of fitness class you can imagine. Boxing, kickboxing, step, Pilates, hip hop, dance, yoga. You name it, I taught it. I completely immersed myself in everything fitness and it felt like the perfect fit.

Here's the not so perfect part...

Between my classes I would secretly go from drug store to drug store and buy up supplies of Syrup of Ipecac. Then I would stop at McDonald's, Taco Bell, any kind of fast food and gorge myself. After that I'd make another stop and put down some ice cream or whatever else I could get. I would literally consume thousands of calories in a single sitting. Then, I would drink a bottle of Syrup of Ipecac and that would cause me to violently throw up. I would throw up to the point of literally vomiting blood. I wanted it that way because that's when I figured that all the food in my system was gone and those "evil" calories couldn't make me fat.

In my late twenties I was doing this three to four times a day and this was my daily routine for years. Yet everyone thought I had it all figured out. That I was the epitome of health. No one knew about my dirty little secret that between my classes I would binge on fast food, and then purge. Then I'd go back and teach another class and cheer people on and say, "Let's get skinny together!" It was such a lie!

The truth was that I was abusing my body on

multiple levels. From what I was eating - and then throwing up - to how I was abusing myself through too much exercise. And perhaps the worst form of abuse was how I talked to myself and beat myself up inside my head.

As I look back, I recognize that I'd never been given the tools on how to manage my inner world. My thoughts, emotions, desires, fears. No one ever teaches you how to deal with that kind of stuff. Yet your inner world contributes more to your overall health, and can bring out a level of hatred and insecurity perhaps more than anything else.

For me, my inner-dialogue was so negative and so destructive that I had completely convinced myself that I was worthless. I was living and working in Los Angeles – the capital of dysfunction - and I was constantly comparing myself to everyone else. Telling myself how inferior I was. This self-loathing and desperation to look a certain way even led me to get liposuction... because in my mind I was just disgusting and I couldn't handle the way I looked.

To put it mildly, my life was a total mess. I was working seventy hours a week, throwing up several times a day, teaching twenty classes a week and abusing myself on all levels – and yet nobody knew it. That's because I knew how to mask what was really going on.

Most of us can do that, right?

We put on masks to convince the world that we're fine when in reality, we're hurting.

"Between classes I would binge on fast food, and then purge. Then I'd teach another class and cheer people on and say, 'Let's get skinny together!' It was such a lie!"

While you may not suffer from the extremes of bulimia and negative self-loathing like I did, I'll bet you've struggled with dieting, exercising and body image at some point in your life. In fact, for most of the women I talk to around the world, this is a daily struggle.

We haven't figured out an effective way to be healthy. We continue to punish our bodies through excessive exercise, crazy dieting and negative self-talk. Or, we just give up and we stop moving our bodies entirely. Then, we overeat or eat things that don't make us feel our best. We allow negative thoughts to dominate our internal conversations. We forget how special and unique we are. We put our needs on the back burner to everyone else's. We lose hope.

That was my life for longer than I'd like to think about – but then I had my awakening and things very quickly took an amazing turn.

===

Dancing is only part of why I love Body Groove. It is the inspirational messages that come along with it. Misty has helped me understand that I am an unique person and that I am okay. I don't fit into anybody's mold. I am learning to love who I am and that I am an okay person.

Grooving has taught me it is okay to take care of myself and do something positive and healthy for myself. It is okay to put me as number one.

I am learning that my way is the right way. Most of all I am setting myself free of all the negative talk in my brain.

Roiann B.

Chapter 2

Fitness Industry Lies

*"Work out because you love your body,
not because you hate it."*

Unknown Author

When I was battling with bulimia, I literally traded my health for my looks, and it almost killed me. However, at the time, I didn't care about that. I just wanted to be thin and didn't think about the long-term consequences of how I was abusing my body. Isn't that how we think and act sometimes when we want to lose weight? Ironically, we're willing to sacrifice our health to "look healthy."

In this quest to look good at all costs we often treat health like it's a destination with a fixed end. It's almost as if we believe that one day we'll simply be deemed "healthy" and that's the end of the whole ordeal. That we can adopt certain practices temporarily to help us lose weight or look better, and then simply abandon these practices once we reach our goal.

This is a huge mistake! It encourages things like dangerous diets and diet supplements, as well as super intense fitness programs that aren't appropriate for most people. Plus, it contributes to a whole host of issues concerning negative body image that leave you feeling like you're not enough.

While it's never good to carry too much excess weight, and there's certainly nothing wrong with having weight loss goals, the fact is, true health encompasses so much more than just your dress size. It's about doing things every day to create a lifestyle that allows you to experience vitality and vibrance. And while this includes things you would normally associate with being healthy, like eating whole foods and exercising, it's also about adopting practices that will allow you to be healthy on the inside.

Think about it like this, I'm sure you've been on a diet at some point in your life. At first this diet probably helped you lose a little weight. But did this diet really make you healthy? Did it set you up for long-term success? More important, did it address any of your inner struggles that contributed to you wanting to lose weight in the first place? Probably not.

For me, part of the reason I made myself throw up after I ate was because I thought it would make me look better. However, there was so much more to my bulimia than just wanting to look good. The truth is, I fooled myself into thinking that if I could look a certain way that everything else in my life would magically be better. Things like my poor body image, my negative inner-dialogue, my low self-esteem. That it would all disappear.

However, rather than my bulimia helping with these things, it just made them worse. It wasn't until I focused on changing my internal thoughts, emotions and habits, and doing what was necessary to get healthy on the inside, that I was able to get healthy on the outside.

But that's not what's being taught in the fitness industry or portrayed in society. Instead, it's about what you look like on the outside, and how quickly you can lose enough weight to rock a bikini. Or, it's the latest "breakthrough" diet that will help you eat whatever you want and still lose incredible amounts of weight. But what about the side effects of these "get-thin-quick" programs? No one ever seems to talk about that. The conversation should be focused on the choices that you can make to ensure lasting health and wellness for the rest of your life, not just for a short period of time.

> *"The fitness industry operates under the assumption that everyone moves the same way. What works for one person will work for another."*

My Dilemma

I was facing a real dilemma. I was a fitness instructor with a crisis of conscious. I had come to the conclusion that the "look-good-at-all-costs" approach to fitness was the worst way to do things. It had not only been detrimental to my health and well-being, but also countless others. I needed to find a more effective way to help myself and my students get healthy. But I was now going to have to fight against an industry that spends billions of dollars convincing people that they are broken and needed fixing. That they're not enough.

As I saw it, there were two major problems with the fitness industry that were preventing people from achieving real long-lasting results.

First, the fitness industry generally doesn't value your individuality. Nowhere is this more apparent than in the structure that it tends to apply to its classes. If you go to gyms and fitness centers all around the world you would see the same kind of classes, taught by the same kind of people, with the same kind of expectations and instructions. These classes emphasize copying a leader rather than moving in a way that makes sense for each individual student. They operate under the assumption that everyone moves the same way and that what works for one person will work for another.

However, when you move your body you should always ask yourself how the movement makes you feel? Is it something that will work for you? Is it right for your body?

These types of questions are typically absent from most exercise classes because the fitness industry doesn't tend to concern itself with something as "trivial" as an individual person's feelings and abilities. And sadly, many fitness instructors are too arrogant to believe that their clients might actually know more about the best way to move their bodies than they do.

Let me assure you, when it comes to your body, no one knows more than you. You are the expert!

My Revelation

Like most every other fitness instructor, my students looked at me and copied what I did. We'd line up in a very regimented fashion and they'd follow everything I told them. Or, at least they would try. Quite often, as soon as many of these students figured out one of the moves I was teaching, I was already onto the next one. It was a constant game of catch-up. My guess is that if you've ever done a fitness class, you can probably relate.

I remember one class in particular where I was really paying attention to my students and trying to figure out how to best help them. What I realized was shocking!

As I looked at my students, I noticed the pain on their faces as they tried to keep up. So many of them were struggling to follow what I was doing. As I watched this more and more I remember thinking how these people really shouldn't be copying me. Their bodies were different than mine and they should move them in a way that was best for them.

However, more than this, I recognized the desperation these people felt to be thin. Their longing to be loved and to feel better about themselves. It was so clear to me. I knew exactly what they were thinking and feeling because I was thinking and feeling the same thing. It didn't matter that I was the teacher and they were the students. Just like me, they were insecure, unsure and vulnerable.

As I was processing this, a surge of empathy came over me and from that moment everything shifted. I realized that the "follow the leader" style of teaching, combined with the mentality that you're broken and need fixing, wasn't going to cut it anymore. Now, I had to figure out something that would. I had to approach teaching differently and I was determined to figure out a better way. A more personal way.

"True beauty is an essence. An understanding of your true worth and value. A liberating state of mind that allows you to be exactly who you are without worrying about what others think, or how they might judge you."

True Health Begins on the Inside

The second major problem with the fitness industry is that in addition to not allowing for creativity or individuality, it focuses almost entirely on a person's outward appearance. Yet, as I've mentioned about my own experience with bulimia, this is the totally wrong way to look at being healthy or beautiful.

When I was throwing up 3-4 times a day I may have looked healthy, or thin on the outside, but I wasn't remotely healthy on the inside. The truth is, I wasn't healthy on the outside either. The constant throwing up depleted my body of much needed nutrients and caused all kinds of problems. I had huge boils on my skin, my hair was falling out and my teeth were decaying. I couldn't go to the bathroom for days at a time. I was a complete mess. I assure you there is so much more to being healthy than just trying to look good.

To be truly healthy you need to begin on the inside, and work your way out. Meaning, you have to cultivate practices in your life that allow your body to function at its best. For me, that meant being more present with the things I was doing. Whether that was how I was exercising, how I was eating, how I was talking to myself, and even how I was interacting with others.

For example, when I was struggling with bulimia, I used to shovel food into my mouth so quickly that I wouldn't even taste it. However, when I decided to be more present with my food, I slowed down and savored every bite. I started asking myself how the food I was eating would make me feel. Was it something that was good for my body? Was it something that I needed?

This practice really changed my perspective on food. It allowed me to stop looking at food as some kind of enemy but as my friend. Now, I no longer feel the urge to binge or mindlessly stuff food into my mouth. I am able to make food choices based on what will make me feel better.

This paradigm shift in how I eat has had a huge impact on me and has transformed my relationship with food. For perhaps the first time in my life, I've stopped dieting and worrying about restricting my calories. Instead, I focus on giving my body what it needs to feel good. Don't get me wrong, I still love cookies. However, if I feel like a cookie, I only eat one or two, rather than the whole batch.

In other areas of my life, I take time for myself each day to think about who I want to be, and the happiness I want to experience. These quiet moments of mediation are extremely powerful as they allow me to recognize my own true worth and beauty, and to reinforce the truth that I am enough. That I can love myself.

You can experience this too.

When you cultivate a healthy inner world, your outer world will almost magically take care of itself. And even though this often means your body will naturally drop unhealthy weight, like it did for me, it's not about achieving a specific size or shape. Instead, it's about an essence. An understanding of your true worth and value. A liberating state of mind that allows you to be exactly who you are without worrying about what others think, or how they might judge you. An intuitiveness about who you are and what your body needs to be truly healthy.

When you stop worrying about what others think so much and give yourself permission to think, move, and act in a way that your body is telling you to, that's when magic can happen. It happened for me and I know can happen for you too.

_____

I have gone from a girl who has hated every workout I have ever tried, to the girl who gets excited to workout when I get home. Knowing that I "can't get it wrong" and hearing "if it doesn't feel good, don't do it" makes all the difference. The music is awesome, the dancing is fun, and most importantly, it's good for the soul. The workshop is amazing as well, helping me to find more of myself. Added bonus, I have lost 30 pounds so far, making myself healthier, not only in weight, but in my entire body. Thank you for creating such an amazing movement.

Misty H.

Chapter 3

The Groove Truths

"Find out who you are and do it on purpose."

- Dolly Parton

Have you ever felt just petrified of being thought of as different or weird?

For me, I was so desperate to fit in that I lived my life doing things in the hope that other people would like me. Or, that they wouldn't think that I was different or weird. Because of this, I never really took the time to think about the things that made me happy, or what I wanted. Instead, I let society do all my thinking for me.

When I finally realized that doing things just to fit in was a recipe for utter misery, I started to explore more about who I was and what I wanted. I knew that I had different qualities and attributes than everyone else but I was too afraid to embrace them. I considered these differences more like a curse than a blessing. However, when I thought about the times in my life when I was truly happy, those were the times when I was doing things that were best suited to my unique personality. Rather than running from these things, I had to embrace them. Otherwise, I would never experience the happiness that I so desperately craved.

> *"You should never judge or criticize yourself because you do things differently than someone else. You're supposed to do things differently. It's what makes you special."*

You have unique talents and characteristics too. Now, you may not think that right now, but I assure you that you do. There are things that make you special. And these things have nothing to do with your size, your looks, your bank account, or how many friends you have on social media. They come from within. The really cool part is that your unique attributes aren't something that make you special in the future, when you've lost weight or look better in a bikini... or any other kind of future. Rather, they make you special right now.

As I began to experiment doing things in a different way, and incorporating my unique skills and attributes more into my life, I developed a set of truths that have come to form the basis for my Body Groove program. I consider these truths to be the very things that have helped me create a happy, healthy life. I refer to these truths as the "Groove Truths" and I've been teaching them to women - and men - all over the world.

Now, even though I say that these truths were developed, they actually came to my mind more like a lightning bolt. They were so clear and loud to me that they were impossible to ignore. And they weren't just vague ideas that I could think about and implement at some point in the future. These were things that I felt compelled to act on immediately. And let me tell you, they have made all the difference.

I want you to experience the liberating power of these Groove Truths, too. So, let's dive right in.

Groove Truth #1:
You are Unique

The first Body Groove Truth is that you are a unique individual. Because of this you're supposed to be different than everyone else, and this is a really good thing.

Think about it like this...

Even though there are nearly seven billion people in the world, no two people are exactly alike. While we share many characteristics, we're all different. The way we look, think, feel, act, move. Because of this, you should never judge yourself or criticize yourself in any way because you do things differently than someone else. You're supposed to do things differently. It's what makes you special. This is especially true when it comes to moving your body.

The concept of moving your own unique way first dawned on me when I was teaching a fitness class. As mentioned, I used to teach a lot of the "follow-the-leader" types of classes where people would line up in rows and just copy everything I showed them.

These classes follow an evolutionary pattern. At first you have a lot of people trying them but after a little while, the only people still coming back are those who are relatively fit, feel coordinated, and are comfortable in a fitness class environment. As you probably know, that's not most people.

In fact, most people would never go to a group fitness class because they don't want to willingly subject themselves to the pain, frustration, and even humiliation that many group classes can cause. Whether it's because they're embarrassed about their size, they don't feel coordinated, or they're not able to follow along, most people tend to avoid these types of classes - especially ones that involve any kind of dancing.

The more I thought about this the more my current style of teaching stopped making sense. First, for many of the reasons mentioned earlier, the people who would benefit the most from coming to my classes simply weren't coming. Second, the people who did come to my classes weren't getting a workout that best suited their body. Instead, they were getting a workout that best suited my body. They'd come to my class and stand in these very structured rows and try to emulate everything I did. No matter what their own personal style of moving or expressing themselves might have been, they were in my class to move exactly like me.

I knew that if I could work with everyone in a one on one manner, I could help them figure out a better way to move their bodies. But I couldn't give that kind of individual attention in a group setting. And sadly, merely copying my movements wasn't going to help these people as much as they hoped it would, or as much as I wanted it too.

Here's what it boils down to...

No one has your body. No one has your structure, your form, your goals, your limitations, or your history. You are unique and you need to move uniquely. Trying to move like someone else just doesn't make sense. It's not smart. Not only could copying someone else actually be dangerous, but also there's something really powerful about learning to be authentically yourself and moving your body in your own unique way.

With this in mind, I started experimenting in my classes and encouraging variations in my student's movement. I wanted to give them permission to be authentic, to be unique, and to be creative. Essentially, I was giving them permission to be themselves. As I did this, I couldn't believe the impact it had on the women in my class. It was remarkable. And it wasn't a physical thing. It was so much deeper than that.

You see, like me, these women were just so tired of punishing themselves to look and act a certain way. And simply giving these women permission to move in a way that felt right for them, was the catalyst for them taking liberties in other areas of their life. All of a sudden they started having more self confidence, doing things they normally wouldn't, and most importantly - accepting and loving their bodies. All because they started to move in a way that felt right for them.

Looking back, this simple yet powerful experiment was the beginning of Body Groove.

"Don't try to follow anyone else's rules. Don't try to follow anyone else's anything. Follow your own intuitive self."

Coming to appreciate your own unique attributes and qualities can sometimes be overwhelming. Many of you have beaten yourself up for so long with such terrible and destructive self-talk, that you may not believe that you're special or unique in any way. I assure you that nothing could be further from the truth. As you continue with me, I will show you how to recognize and embrace all of your remarkable and amazing gifts.

For now, please accept that because you are unique, you should be different, and this makes you special. So, let yourself be different. Don't try to follow anyone else's patterns. Don't try to follow anyone else's rules. Don't try to follow anyone else's anything.

Follow your own intuitive self. The deepest desires of your heart and what you want to do.

I'm currently doing the Body Groove 30 day challenge. It's helping me BIG time to work through old emotions and feelings, and the dancing afterwards is SO freeing. The meditation and self awareness exercises are extremely beneficial, something I had a hard time with before. Being constantly reminded that "you can't get it wrong," and "whatever feels right for you IS right" is KEY. It immediately reminds me to shed the negative thoughts sneaking in.

My 9 year old daughter joins me often and the lessons she is learning about loving herself are so comforting knowing she is soon going to be subjected to the world's views of what is "pretty". She has also reminded me in key moments (ie. bathing suit shopping) that it doesn't matter what anyone else thinks and that I look beautiful.

I will forever be a Groover. I could not be more thankful that I came across Body Groove. It is life changing!

Shannon S.

Chapter 4

No One Cares

"You probably wouldn't worry about what people think of you if you could know how seldom they do!"

Olin Miller

You've heard it before. The idea that you shouldn't care about what others think. That you should just be yourself and do things your way.

While this sounds great - and it is - it's actually really difficult to put into practice. Whether it's the way you look, what you say, or how you act, no one wants to feel embarrassed or uncomfortable. However, is your fear of embarrassment really worth all the attention you give it?

When I had my "awakening", I realized that I'd spent my whole life doing everything for other people.

The clothes I wore, the car I drove, the area I lived in... even my job. Everything about my life was done to keep up a certain "acceptable" appearance. In fact, my whole sense of importance and self-worth was dependent on making sure others approved of my choices.

It's crazy to think about now, but I experienced severe anxiety about the possibility of losing the approval of others. Or, doing something that might bring some undue attention to myself. This mindset even extended to people I didn't know or have a relationship with. Heaven forbid I did something that someone else might think is weird or bizarre. I just couldn't stand the thought that someone might think less of me. Can you relate?

But here's the problem when you live your life just trying to please others, and being afraid of what they might think of you. The very things that make you special and unique become dormant. All of your amazing characteristics and your true personality traits get hidden from those around you. Plus, it stifles your creativity and imagination, and it prevents you from achieving your potential. This is true in every area of your life. Your work, your relationships, your health and wellness... everything!

Just imagine if some of the world's greatest innovators, artists, or leaders, constantly worried about what others thought. We may not have some of the greatest technology, music, literature, art, or so many other things that make our lives so much better. It's the same with you. If you're constantly worried about what others think, you too may never accomplish your greatest work.

"While you might think others are concerned with how you look or what you do, they're really only concerned about themselves."

Just as quickly as I came to the realization that my life choices were made to gain the acceptance of others, I likewise realized that nobody really cared about me and my hang-ups. And that's the big secret that no one ever tells you! Nobody actually cares what you look like. What you wear, where you live, what kind of car you drive, if you have a six-pack, or the size of your butt. No one cares!

Why?

Because they're so completely absorbed with themselves and their own issues that they simply don't have time to worry about you and your issues! And that's the next Body Groove Truth... No one cares what you look like.

Groove Truth #2:
No One Cares What You Look Like

Let's suppose you saw someone you don't know doing something weird, or looking different to what you think is acceptable. How much consideration did you really give this person before you bought your attention back to yourself? Probably not very much. And if you're not giving much attention to those around you, then it stands to reason that they're not thinking about you either. You only think they are.

To prove this to yourself, the next time you go out, pay attention to the people around you and how they act. You'll quickly notice that they aren't worried about you or anyone else. They're only worried about themselves. How they look. How they act. How their latest selfie turned out and how many likes it received. While you might think others are concerned with how you look or what you do, they're really only concerned about themselves and how they think others are judging them.

Sadly, prior to coming to this realization, I had been killing myself trying to impress others. Worrying about what they might think of me. I was literally losing sleep thinking about people looking at my butt and thinking it wasn't perfect. Not only was this just completely exhausting, but it was also an absolute waste of time and energy.

However, when I really embraced the idea that no one cares what I look like, it completely changed my life. First, the need to gain the approval of others completely left me. I can't even begin to tell you how incredibly liberating this was. It immediately allowed me to experience an inner peace that I hadn't felt for years. This allowed so much of the chaos and turmoil inside of my head to disappear. My stress and anxiety levels went down too. All because I stopped worrying about what I thought others were thinking about me.

Second, when you're not obsessing over how to live your life to impress others, it frees up so much space in your mind. With this "space", I was able to unleash a level of creativity that I had never experienced. Things were coming to my mind all the time and it was so exciting. It was like my life was now a blank canvas, ready for me to create my own masterpiece. All because I stopped worrying about what others might think, took the time to figure out what was going to be best for me, and started listening to my own intuition.

Just imagine what your life would be like if instead of going about your day trying to always please others, you had the freedom to be yourself, and do the things that give you the most happiness. I can assure you, it can have truly dramatic results.

"When you free yourself to move in a way that's right for your body, the floodgates open and your authentic, creative self will emerge."

When you stop worrying about what others think, you'll see how doing things your own way can free you both mentally and physically. This will allow you to experience so much happiness in your life. And not just for you, but also the people around you as well.

What if Someone Does Care About What You Look Like? (Or at you least you think they do.)

It's easy to say, "No one cares what you look like," but it takes time and practice to really embrace this truth. With that said, don't get me wrong. There will always be judgmental people in the world that put others down in an attempt to make themselves feel better.

Even the most judgmental people really don't care what you look like or what you're doing. They're only concerned about themselves and their own problems and worries. But let's suppose this wasn't the case and someone really was concerned with how you look – is that really something you need to worry about?

Absolutely not!

You have zero control over how others think and act. If their life is so meaningless to warrant them passing judgement on you, that's something you just don't have to worry about. Other people's opinions of you are irrelevant. All that matters is what you think about yourself.

If you think about it, they're the ones who are stewing in judgmental thoughts. How awful must it be to carry that?

Six months ago I was on the sofa, unhappy with myself and my lack of motivation. I started doing Body Groove and I worked up from dancing to 1-2 groove songs a day, to doing whole segments, 3-4 days a week. I've now lost weight and I feel amazing.

Today I'm moving, I'm dancing all the time. My blood sugar is under better control, the arthritis I have in my left ankle, knee, hip, and low back is much less prevalent...and I'm happier. Which is my FAVORITE result. I tell everyone about Misty and Body Groove!

Dana C.

Chapter 5

Do it Your Way

"You have your way. I have my way. As for the right way,
the correct way, and the only way, it does not exist."

Friedrich Wilhelm Nietzsche

If you ever get the chance to watch a dance fitness class at a gym, don't watch the teacher. Instead, watch the people participating. The teacher is doing a routine they've probably done hundreds of times, and the students are trying to keep up. Inevitably, the students are almost always a couple of steps behind the instructor.

If you've ever done a fitness class like this you can probably relate. The moment you get a move down you light up and it feels really good. But then the instructor goes on to the next move and you're out of sync again. When you finally catch up to that move, you experience that wave of excitement again, only to have the instructor move on to the next move. It's a constant game of catch up. And while it can be really frustrating not doing the choreography perfectly, that's not the biggest problem with these types of classes.

When it comes to moving your body, if you're trying to follow someone else, like a fitness instructor, your attention naturally goes to what they're doing. If you're constantly staring at them and trying to copy them - or catch up to them - you can't pay attention to your own body and what it needs. You won't be able to discover what your individual capabilities are. And you won't be able to explore the depths of what your body can do. Exercising by merely copying someone else's moves won't allow you to be fully present in your own body and recognize what it needs.

"When you move in a way that feels unique to you, you're going to activate all these different parts of yourself - both mind and body - that other workouts can't."

If you're going to put in the effort to workout, you might as well do something that's going to be best for your body. And that's what the next Groove Truth is all about.

Groove Truth #3:
Your Way is the Right Way

Because you are unique (Groove Truth #1), you were designed to do things a certain way. That's especially true when it comes to moving your body. While we all have the same basic make-up, that doesn't mean we're all supposed to move the same way. That's because you have ceratin capabilities and limitations that are unique to you. Your endurance, flexibility, stamina, past injuries, your likes and dislikes, genetics, and so many other things that contribute to figuring out the best way to move your body. Because of this, rather than merely copying someone - who designed a workout for themselves - when you move, you should explore moving in a way that feels right for your body. But how exactly do you do this?

When I first encouraged my students to be creative in the way they moved, many of them looked at me in a very confused way. They'd been so condi-tioned to only follow the leader in a fitness setting, that they didn't quite understand what I wanted them to do. However, it didn't take long for them to embrace what I was asking. In fact, I was amazed at how quickly they were able to find their own unique way of moving. Within just minutes, every person in my class was doing something different. They were all moving their own way and exploring what felt right for them. It was such a beautiful sight.

This experience is one that I've seen this play out over and over again, all around the world. No matter who it's with, or what experience a person has, when you give someone permission to move freely, they just do it. Look at a baby when they hear music. They just move in whatever way that feels natural. It's an innate response and it never leaves you. That's why finding your own unique way to move is as easy as turning the music on and going for it. You just have to go for it!

You Can't Get it Wrong

When you trust your body to move in a way that feels right for you, even though that will be different from everybody else, your body will naturally do things the way that it was designed to. Meaning, that when you do it your way - you can't get it wrong.

Let me repeat that because it's really important. When you move your way, you can't get it wrong.

However, when you are just following the way

someone else moves, it limits you to whatever their limitations are, and pigeon holes you to their level of creativity and expression. Not that you can't draw inspiration or ideas from others. Rather, it's that so much can open up to you when you start to trust your inner voice and move in a way that feels right for your body. And you'll only know what your right way is, when you try.

So, let yourself be different. Embrace your uniqueness. Trust your intuition. Let yourself be weird and crazy. You'll discover things about yourself that will blow your mind when you simply give yourself permission to be unique.

I promise you... Your way is the right way!

Beware of Fear-Restricted Movement

While moving in a way that's right for you can be extremely liberating, it can also be scary. Sometimes even when you're in your own home, by yourself, when no one is watching, you can hold back because you're afraid of what others might think.

Isn't that crazy?

Even when no one is watching, you can still succumb to "fear-restricted movement." This can totally stifle your creativity and ultimately prevent you from reaching your goals. And it's not just in the way you move. Fear can prevent you from achieving your goals in other areas of your life either too. Because of this, you've got to follow your own unique path, even though it might terrify you.

Remember. Because no one actually cares what you look like (Groove Truth #2), you really do have the freedom to move, act, think in the way that feels right to you.

"Life has ups and downs. But you can choose to be miserable and sad. Or, you can choose to stand on your own two feet, and be a warrior and champion of your own life."

Much like all of the Groove Truths, coming to appreciate the idea that your way is the right way can take time. So, start with the way you move. Go somewhere by yourself, turn on the music - or a Body Groove workout - and start to experiment with the way you move. You'll quickly prove to yourself that not only are you more creative than you think, but also that nobody actually cares what you look like. That's because no one's actually looking. No one's judging you. It's you judging yourself. If you can come to accept this, you will no longer be a slave to fear-restricted movement. This will unleash your creativity and allow you to express yourself in a way that is right for you.

When you move in a way that feels unique to your body, you're going to activate all these different parts of yourself - both mind and body - that other "follow-the-leader" workouts can't. You'll be able to explore your full range of motion, strength and flexibility. To express yourself in a fun, creative manner that constantly challenges you. To understand the needs and limitations of your body. And and to appreciate your body and all of its amazing capabilities and wonders. And best of all, you can't get it wrong.

Best of all, this doesn't just apply to moving. When you do things your way, or when you listen to your intuition, you can't get life wrong either. So many of us think there's a right way to do life and a wrong way. Even worse, we compare our lives to others and foolishly think that they have it all figured out and a handle on all their problems. But this just isn't true. Hardly anyone has it figured out. Everyone has problems. However, in my experience, the people who are the happiest, most fulfilled, and have the best handle on life and their problems, are those who listen to their gut and follow their instincts.

Viva La Mexico

Coming to the realization that I had to follow my intuition was something that began with the way I taught my fitness classes. But it didn't stop there. About 10 years ago I sold everything I owned, and moved from my beautiful apartment in Beverly Hills to Mexico.

At the time, everybody told me that I was crazy. They tried to warn me how dangerous it was there, and how it was a mistake for me to turn my back on my career that I'd spent years building. But I knew for myself that I needed to pursue a different path. To really follow what was in my gut despite what anyone else was saying. So, I trusted my inner voice and did what I needed to do for me, even though it looked different than what everyone else was doing, or telling me. Yes, it was scary and I wasn't sure how it was going to turn out. But, giving up my identity was the very thing that helped me find myself. Even though I only had what was in my two suitcases, the quality of my life went through the roof. My happiness skyrocketed and the past ten years have been the most rewarding, eye-opening, creative, fulfilling, productive, lovely years of my life.

Now, by no means do you have to sell everything you own and move to Mexico, or anything even like that. But there is something inside of you. Something you want to do, or some way you want to live or feel, or express yourself. You want to experience certain things that are unique to you and to live a life that is full and purpose and meaning. Sure, life has ups and downs. That's the way it goes. But you can choose to be miserable and sad. Or, you can choose to stand on your own two feet, and be a warrior and champion of your own life. You can't get this wrong. It's just your choice and how you want to live and what you want to do. Your way is the right way.

Whatever capabilities you have, whatever restrictions you might be dealing with, whatever it is that you're working with, it doesn't matter. Play with it. Be fun with it. See what you can do. What feels great and what feels awful. Figure out how every part of your body moves. Let it be weird. Let it not make sense. Let it look silly. Embarrass yourself! When you do it your way, it is the right way and it's the only way that will allow you to find your own vibrant health.

I'm 53 years old and several years ago I lost my ability to walk. My husband had to take me to the bathroom and everything. I was in significant pain every day. I got diagnosed with an autoimmune disorder. Medication helped a little, but then I had side effects to deal with. I finally got tired of being sick and tired. I decided I was going to take my life back as much as I possibly could.

I cleaned up my diet to make sure I had good fuel for my body to heal itself. Then, I discovered Body Groove. I started out with 2 routines a week. As I got stronger, I increased the number of routines I was able to do. My pain level decreased in a major way. My rheumatologist can't believe the turn around in my health. I was practically bedridden, and now I dance. I'm even able to jump and skip. As a matter of fact, I just removed popcorn ceiling and refinished the ceiling in my bathroom all by MYSELF.

This program was a life saver. Never before had I ever been encouraged to modify movement. I was always made to feel that I was less than if I didn't copy the instructor exactly. Guess what? I'm a year into Body Groove, and I no longer have to modify anything. As a bonus, I've gone from a size 20 to a size 12. Take that autoimmune disease!

Laurie V.

Chapter 6

No One Can Do it For You

"The moment you take responsibility for everything in your life is the moment you can change anything in your life."

-Hal Elrod

Growing up, I was convinced that someone was going to come and rescue me. From the stories I've been told, the books I've read, the movies I've watched. I fully expected a knight in shining armor to ride in on his white horse and give me the ultimate wedding, a beautiful home, and an amazing life. But more than the fairy-tale romance, this person was also someone who was going to fix me and take care of me. To solve all of my problems. To make me thin and healthy. To create my dreams for me. To make me happy and to love me. No matter what it was that I needed, I was just going to sit back and someone else was going to do everything for me.

When I finally realized that this someone, who I had waited my whole life for, wasn't coming, it was a real turning point. Reluctantly, I woke up to the fact that there's no knight in shining armor who is coming to rescue me. No one's going to come and make me like myself. Nobody's going to come and live my dreams for me. Nobody's going to be happy for me. Everything I want out of life is my responsibility to achieve. Nobody else's. I know that's harsh, but it's true.

Groove Truth #4:
No One Can Do it for You

For most of my life I had been waiting for something outside of me, or someone, to make me happy. To take care of me and whatever needs I had. But the fact is, no one can actually do any of these things for you.

If you want to dance authentically and creatively, no one can do that for you...

If you want to develop a meditation practice and a more peaceful inner world for yourself, no one can do that for you...

If you want to be happy and content, to live a life of meaning and purpose, no one can do that for you...

If you want to get healthy by eating good foods and exercising more, no one can that for you!

No one can do any of these things for you. But we often think they can and put all of our unreal expectations upon them. We make it their job to make our lives better and to make us happy. News flash! It's not up to them. It's your responsibility and yours alone.

When you put your happiness, or your joy, or your inner peace, or anything you really want on someone or something outside of yourself, it becomes extremely vulnerable. You are no longer in control of your destiny and you're at the whim of what happens to you every day.

Think about it like this...

As women, we have a tendency to be a little more emotional than men, which is fine. I think it's beautiful that we're this way. But if you're not in touch with managing these emotions and thoughts, than every day can be like a roller coaster. You're up. You're down. You're sad. You're happy. You're all over the place. Your day hinges on what someone else says, how they look at you, or what they do.

Stop giving others that kind of power over you! Don't let the everyday circumstances of your day dictate your outlook. Come to terms with the idea that no one is coming to rescue you, but that you must rescue yourself. Be responsible for your own happiness and everything else in your life. You're the only one who can.

"There's always going to be things that are going to irritate you, but it's up to you how you want to respond. It's up to you whether you want to react and feed into it."

Your Blue Print for Happiness

One of the easiest ways I was able to start taking action in my own life was by focusing on things that bought me happiness and fulfillment. I quickly noticed how these things weren't over the top or extravagant. Instead, they were actually very simple. Like taking a yoga class from a teacher who really helps me connect to myself. Going salsa dancing. Going for a bike ride. Reading. Meditating. Grooving. Socializing and connecting authentically with other people.

In fact, I even made a list of these simple things that allow me to experience so much happiness. And as simple as it sounds, this list became a blueprint for my happiness. That's because once I had my list, I intentionally looked for opportunities to do more of these "list-things" in my life.

What about you? What things bring you joy?

It could be a walk in the park, or a walk on the beach. It could be a talk with a friend or loved one. It could be a great cup of coffee in the morning. Whatever it is that brings you joy is your road map to happiness. Your job is to figure out how to fill your day with as much of these things as possible.

Now, keep in mind, there's always going to be things that are going to irritate and bother you, but it's up to you how you want to respond to these annoyances. It's up to you whether you want to react and feed into it. Or, you can choose to spend your precious life, energy and time doing things that bring you joy. After all... no one can do it for you.

Healthy Selfish

Have you ever noticed in your life how much you give, and give, and give? You give everyone else your time, your attention, your admiration. Especially as women. So often your needs take a back seat to the needs of others. Your spouse, your partner, your kids, your work, your friends. It can leave you feeling depleted, frustrated, and sometimes even angry.

This is a backwards way of trying to be happy. Instead, you should be giving your time and attention to yourself, well before you give it to others. You should be the number one thing on your to-do list every single day.

Why?

Because you are worthy of your time. You are worthy of your attention. You deserve to fulfill your needs, achieve your goals, and to be happy. Besides, as we've just discussed, no one's going to do it for you. You have to do it for yourself. If you want to get healthy, if you want to be happy, if you want to accomplish something, it's going to require putting yourself first. In fact, it's essential that you put yourself first.

Now, please don't misunderstand the notion of putting yourself first in these situations as being selfish. Instead, I like to think of it as being healthy selfish.

Being "healthy selfish" requires that you focus on the things that will allow you to be the best version of yourself. It allows you to create a peaceful inner world. It gives you a foundation where you can create change if you so desire. It allows you to discover your purpose, and to pursue the things that are going to bring you the most joy. It gives you the opportunity and time to invest in yourself every single day, knowing that you're worthy of it.

Plus, when your needs are fulfilled, and you've

given yourself the time and attention you deserve, you can be the best version of yourself for others too. You can be a better spouse. A better mom. A better worker. A better listener... A better everything.

You can be more compassionate. More caring. Move giving. More loving. More empathetic... More everything.

Yes. Some people may resent you for focusing on yourself first. However, it's really important to ignore these voices because in order to be the kind of person you want to be for others, you first need to take care of yourself. Once your needs and wants are met, that's when you can more easily take care of those who depend on you.

Remember, you are worthy of your time, your attention, your affection, and your love.

After being a stay at home/work from home Mom who sat in a chair for most of the day for 25+years...I admit I didn't feel very well but didn't know what was wrong. I tried over 2 years to diet and exercise and always felt like that damn scale mocked me. I'd lose a couple, gain a couple, up and down, and still felt exhausted, overwhelmed and just hating life. I was severely depressed, having multiple panic attacks, and was having some serious health issues, couldn't sleep, and just felt terrible all the time.

Then I saw Misty. I ordered Body Groove and couldn't wait to get going. Funny thing is I thought it was just fun dancing, had no clue about the workshop! I signed up for the on-demand and got started on the workshop. I finished it in 3 days and went right into the 30 day challenge. OMG! What a difference in my life! I feel amazing!! I have lost weight, am eating right, dancing, doing water workouts, but those are actually just side effects of the real change.

I am so much more at peace! The panic attacks still come, but I can dance through them now! The tears still come but I start to move and they stop. I meditate, dance, breathe, and even was inspired in one meditation to paint! Body Groove is life changing.

Caren M.

Chapter 7

You Must Apply It

"It doesn't matter who you are, where you come from. The ability to triumph begins with you – always."

Oprah Winfrey

So far we've talked about the first four Groove Truths: You are unique. No one cares what you look like. Your way is the right way. No one can do it for you.

Now, as life changing as these Truths can be, they can't help you until you actually apply them. They're just principles. Good ideas. In order for them to be of benefit, you must put them into practice. And that leads us to the final Groove Truth.

Groove Truth #5:
You Must Apply it

The fifth Groove Truth is all about taking action. You doing the work that's required to make a difference in your life. You see, just knowing that you're unique doesn't do you any good if you don't express your uniqueness...

Just knowing that no one really cares what you look like doesn't mean anything if you're unwilling to look, move and act in a way that feels right to you...

Being told that your way is the right way doesn't help you express your creativity or act on your intuition if you continue to only follow others...

Understanding that you're the only one who can make yourself happy, eat healthy, exercise, and so many other things, doesn't help if you're not going to actually do these things. You must take action.

By putting the Groove Truths into practice you can more readily accomplish your goals and experience the happiness in your life that you deserve. If you don't take the necessary action steps, these Truths are just ideas that won't ever amount to anything. That won't help you have a better life. That won't get you to where you want to be. You have to take action.

Now, implementing these Truths doesn't have

to be difficult. What's so beautiful about the Groove Truths is they can be practiced all the time in so many simple ways.

The clothes you wear. The people you associate with. How you choose to move when you exercise. How you spend your free time. What music you listen to. What movies or television you watch. The podcasts you engage with. Even who you choose to follow on social media. You can find your own voice and be your own person in all of these things. You can even apply these Truths to trivial things like how you prepare and drink your coffee in the morning. No matter what it is in your life, you can practice listening to your inner voice and taking the steps to follow that voice.

"I finally was like, 'I'm going to stand up for the life that I want to live. I am enough and I'm going to start living accordingly.' "

When you start following your intuition and doing things that will make you happy, here's something to consider. There's nothing to master. Nothing to ever get 100% right. Nothing that you ever have to totally figure out. If you decide to meditate it's something you can practice but nothing you're required to be perfect at. The same when you dance. Just have fun with it. You don't need to master how to dance, you just need to move your own way and do what feels right. And this is true with just about everything. Rather than thinking you need to be perfect at what you're doing, just always try to follow your voice and do it your way. And most of all, have fun doing it. Otherwise, what's the point?

A Super Easy Way to Apply the Groove Truths

When the Groove Truths first came to me, the easiest and most natural way for me to implement them in my life was on the dance floor.

Just think about the principles that make up the Groove Truths. You are unique. No one cares what you look like. Your way is the right way. No one can do it for you. All of these can be perfectly applied (Groove Truth #5) when you dance. In fact, it was applying these Truths while dancing that led to the creation of my Body Groove program.

With Body Groove you can be totally unique. You can dance without having to care about what others think. You can move in a way that is right for you. No one can do it for you.

But it doesn't stop there.

The courage and confidence you build while

applying these Truths while Grooving, can transcend into other areas of your life. This includes your relationships, your work, your mind set, your food choices, the way you talk to yourself, your attitude about life, and practically everything else you do.

I cannot tell you how many people have shared how their lives changed when they started Grooving. All of a sudden they found themselves with more confidence, loving themselves, taking risks, wearing different clothes, doing things they've always wanted to do but were afraid to try. Even their relationships with their spouses, children and friends... they all improve. That's how powerful these Truths can be. It starts on the dance floor, by somehow magically carries over into every area of your life.

WARNING! *Crazy Lady Dancing*

Let me give you an example of how I like to apply the Groove Truths.

I love to put my air pods in and dance by myself. But here's the catch. I like to do this on the beach. Which means I'm typically being watched - or stared at - by others. What they see is this "crazy" woman completely rocking out on the beach in her own world.

While I'm aware that almost everyone on the beach is looking at me, at the end of the day, I know these people really don't care what I look like. While they might get a chuckle every now and again, they will go on with their lives and not give me a second thought.

However, what I get out of doing this is so much more than the people watching me. It's not just about moving my body and getting my Groove on. It's also about doing something that makes me feel amazing and confident. I can't even tell you how ready I am to take on the world after dancing on the beach like this. If I can dance in front of strangers and look "crazy," I can do pretty much anything.

If I didn't practically apply the principle that no one cares what I look like, then I'd be the one deprived of an opportunity to be happy. I'd be the one who didn't experience a boost to her confidence, or the one who didn't get to express herself creatively.

Now, I'm not suggesting that you need to dance on the beach in front of strangers. That's what I like to do. Besides, that might not make you happy. Instead, you have to figure out what you want to do to apply the Groove Truths in your life. And keep in mind, these things can be really can be simple, like sitting for a minute or two in the morning to breathe and think about how good your life is. Buying yourself flowers from time to time. Taking an extra long bath. Going for a walk. Listening to a podcast of someone you admire.

Taking a local college class or workshop that interests you, or any number of really simple things.

The bottom line is that I want you to stand on your own two feet and be the warrior and champion for your own life. That's what I finally did. I was like, "I'm gonna stand up for myself. I'm going to stand up for my health. I'm going to stand up for my happiness. I'm going to stand up for the life that I want to live. I am enough and I'm going to start living accordingly."

You can do the same and it really can be easy. All it takes is just a little bit of practice every day.

This is a huge year for me. In a couple of weeks I turn 60. How on earth did that happen? I've long had issues with weight, the scale, dieting. Then, about 6 months ago I saw that one of my daughter's friends "liked" a page called Body Groove on Facebook. I looked at the post but never went any further.

Don't you know, like some secret message, it kept on appearing on my Facebook page - I ultimately clicked on it - saw some folks dancing WITHOUT SNEAKERS!!! I was immediately mesmerized.

It took another couple of months for me to sign up for the 30 day challenge and I was hooked. I. Love. Body. Groove. In my years of trying to figure out what exercise was best for me - it's cold, I can't walk. It's raining, I can't walk. Kettle bells, ugh. Gym equipment, yawn. But dance?!?!? I am a child of the 70's! I love dancing! And I can look silly (quite well I might add) but I've been grooving 6 days a week for almost 3 months now. No excuses. Just dance.

Thank you for what you do for people like me. You made something as boring (in my mind) as routine exercise into something absolutely freeing and enjoyable and a little gritty! I'm heading straight for 60 with sass and grit and groove.

Susan J.

Chapter 8

Discover Your Groove 30-Day Challenge

"Challenges make you discover things about yourself that you never really knew."

Cicely Tyson

I truly believe that once you begin implementing the Groove Truths that your life will radically change for the better. However, knowing the Truths and living them are two different things. They will take patience and practice. Perhaps years to fully embrace. So, as you try to implement these Truths, just know that it'll take some time. Yes, you'll see immediate results but it is a journey.

Perhaps the easiest place to start applying the Groove Truths is in the way you move.

Here's why...

I created Body Groove to be an alternative to the traditional "follow-the-leader" types of exercise. These other exercises are often too painful, too stressful, and they don't allow you to move in a way that's right for your body. Plus, I found from teaching so many of these kinds of classes that they just weren't giving people the results they wanted. Body Groove changes that.

While it's low-impact and stress-free, the best thing about it is that I give you a basic move or two, and then encourage you to make each move your own. You get to experiment with how you move your body and have the freedom to move it completely different to me and to everyone else. Whatever is right for you.

While this is extremely liberating - and fun - it can also be a little intimidating too. You're probably not used to doing exercise without a rigid structure. You may be afraid to dance and move your body creatively. However, don't worry about that. I'll show you how to do it and make it so that it's not difficult.

When you free yourself to move in a way that's right for your body, the floodgates open and your authentic, creative self will emerge. Your body will naturally and effortlessly move toward a healthy state, both inside and out.

The Discover Your Groove 30-Day Challenge

I want you to apply the Groove Truths in your life, especially in the way you exercise. I want you to flex the muscle that nobody cares. Flex the muscle that your way is the right way. Flex the muscle that no one can do this for you and flex the muscle that you are absolutely a unique individual and that you should be different.

The Discover Your Groove Challenge is where you get to practice all of the Groove Truths. But more than that, I'm going to take you for 30 days through my workshop and favorite dances. I'm going to be your personal coach and friend for the 30 days and we're going to dance together, journal, meditate, and other little activities to enrich your physical, emotional and mental wellness.

Together, we're going to go explore deep into who you are, and figure out how to nurture your inner world. Your thoughts, feelings, emotions... the way you talk to yourself. That's because the narrative you create in your inner-world eventually becomes your reality in your outer-world.

At the end of our 30 days together I promise

that your life will be so enriched and you will be on the path to a happy, healthy life. Your best life.

So join me today. I know you're going to love it.

To begin your 30 day Discover Your Groove Challenge you'll need to go to link below and sign up. Here's the link...

www.bodygroove.com/30daychallenge

Tips for making the most out of your 30 Day Discover Your Groove Challenge:

- Take one day at a time.
- Read the daily instructions, watch the workshop videos, do the groove workout.
- If you miss a day or two, just pick it back up when you're ready.
- Don't rush it. It's not a race to complete this so try and make each day really count.
- Keep a journal.
- Have fun.

Day 1 - Your Ideal Life

I want you to ask yourself the very question that I asked myself all those years ago when I was laying on my bathroom floor covered in vomit and blood.

"Is this as good as it gets?"

With this question in mind, I want you to start thinking about the things in your life that you want to improve. Perhaps you could start by identifying broad areas of your life that need your attention. For example, you might see that your eating habits need to change, or that your mind-set could be more positive.

As you think about these things try to be as specific as possible. And don't be afraid to take a look at ALL areas of your life. Think about your relationships, your work, your finances, your habits. Don't let any area of your life go un-examined.

Next, I want you to divide all these "improvements" into two categories: things you can change, and things you can't.

You see, there are some things in your life that you cannot change, no matter what you do. You can't change your genetics, or your history. That's not to say that it's irrational to wish that those things were different. I've inherited some health challenges that I wish I didn't have. And, there are some very painful things in my past that I wish I could erase. However, no matter how much I wish those things were different or didn't happen, there is nothing I can do to change them. I have found though, as I've focused on the areas in my life that I can change, I've realized that I actually have more power and influence than I thought. I believe you will come to this conclusion too.

So, to get started, go to the link below, or login to your Body Groove On-Demand account and get started on your first day's workshop and dance videos.

Here's the link to today's activities. Remember to watch the workshop first and then come back and do today's assignment. Oh, and you can do today's Groove's at any time. Enjoy!

www.bodygroove.com/day1

ASSIGNMENT FOR DAY 1:

Identify and write down the things in your life that you want to work on. Take as much time as you need and be specific. And, examine all areas of your life, both big and small. Next, I want you to categorize your list into things you can change, and things you can't. Over the coming days, we're going to take steps to make changes in the areas that you can control.

What are some of areas of your life that you'd like to work on? When you've listed these, place a check beside the things that you can change, and a cross besides the things you can't.

_____

_____

_____

_____

_____

_____

_____

_____

_____

_____

_____

_____

_____

_____

_____

_____

_____

_____

_____

_____

_____

_____

Day 2 - Your Life Answers

I hope you had the chance to think about yesterday's activity and to write down the things in your life that you'd like to work on. Today, we're going to talk about the importance, AND the limitations of coaches, advisors and mentors.

Like many of you, I enjoy watching figure skating in the Olympics. As someone who never felt at home on an ice rink, I'm amazed by what world class skaters can accomplish. In thinking about this, consider how important it is for these skaters to have coaches to help and guide them. In fact, it's often having the right coach that can make a figure skater's career. But these coaches aren't helpful because they have more ice skating skills, or more ice skating experience. In fact, every Olympic figure skater is coached by someone who is less skilled than they are.

The real value of coaches isn't that they have all the answers to your questions, or that they've already solved all your problems. The most helpful coaches are the ones who can help you better understand YOURSELF, your abilities, your weaknesses, your blind spots, and your opportunities. As your Body Groove coach, that's what I want to do for you.

Of course, I don't have all the answers for you,

I'm just here as a guide to help you figure things out for yourself. The Discover Your Groove Challenge isn't about copying all MY answers, or copying MY life. Instead, it's about coming up with the answers that are best for you and your life.

So, with that in mind, watch today's workshop videos where I talk about coaching and how it can best help you. Afterwards, I'll lead you through your daily groove.

Here's today's link...

www.bodygroove.com/day2

ASSIGNMENT FOR DAY 2:

Look at your list from yesterday (or think about it if you didn't write anything down) and pick one thing that you'd like to focus on. Now, think about how YOU can come up with some answers or solutions to what area you picked. Really take some time to ponder how things can be better or different. Use that big, beautiful brain you have figure out the things that will help you have the life you deserve. The answers are inside of you and will mean so much more when you discover them.

Pick something from yesterday's list that you'd like to focus on making better. What can you do to make an impact in this area of your life?

_____

_____

_____

_____

_____

_____

_____

_____

_____

_____

_____

_____

_____

_____

_____

_____

_____

_____

Day 3 - Let Yourself be Weird

For today's coaching session, we're simply going to dance to a variety of routines from the Body Groove collection. However, I'd like for you to pay attention to one dance in particular. It's called "Guilt" and it's from my House Party video collection. This special routine is a great workout that will do wonders for your strength and flexibility, but there's also a hidden challenge in it. In this workout, I specifically ask you to be...weird. That's right, weird.

Weird can mean lots of things. Your definition of weird is going to be different than everyone else's. So, you'll need to figure out what it looks like for you.

Now, while you're grooving to the "Guilt" routine, or after, I want you to ask yourself the following questions...

1. Do you find it difficult to be weird, even if it's just for a brief moment, and in the privacy of your own home?

2. If you do have a hard time being weird - and almost everyone does - why is that? What makes it so difficult?

Remember, I don't have all your answers. You'll need to explore this for yourself. But I will tell you, the less I worry about what other people might think of me, and the more I simply ALLOW myself to be myself, the more I'm able to express my own creativity. Or, the more my "weird" comes out. This is a truly liberating feeling. I want you to experience it too.

So, go and do my "Guilt" workout, and then grab your pen and paper and write down your thoughts about being weird.

Here's today's link...

www.bodygroove.com/day3

ASSIGNMENT FOR DAY 3:

As you dance today, I want you to be as weird, or creative, as you possibly can. Really allow yourself to explore what your body can do and don't be afraid to be go places you've never been. I guarantee, the more weird you allow yourself to be, the more fun you'll have.

If you found it difficult to be "weird" in your Groove today, write down what's holding you back. What steps could you take to overcome this?

_____

_____

_____

_____

_____

_____

_____

_____

When you were able to let go and be "weird," how did that make you feel? Did you surprise yourself in any way? Are there other areas of your life that you can be "weird?" If so, how will this benefit you?

_____

_____

_____

_____

_____

_____

_____

_____

Day 4 - The Healing Power of Dance

There's a saying that goes, "In this world nothing can be said to be certain, except death and taxes." I'd like to add two things to this list of life certainties. Stress and anxiety. They're an unavoidable fact of life. And while there are lots of things we can and should do to reduce the stress in our lives, we can never get rid of it completely. The question then becomes, "how do you deal with it?"

We learn all kinds of coping skills for stress and anxiety as we go through life. Some are these can be really destructive, like drug or alcohol abuse, or my old "favorite" - binge eating and bulimia. Others are relatively harmless, like eating ice cream, vegging in front of the TV, or mindlessly scrolling through your social media feed. While these coping methods never actually reduce our stress or anxiety, they at least distract us for a while.

In today's Body Groove workshop, we talk about a coping skill that really does alleviate stress and anxiety. Plus, it's actually good for you too. I'm talking about dancing! Dancing can be the perfect way to help you release stress and decrease anxiety.

Here's today's link...

www.bodygroove.com/day4

ASSIGNMENT FOR DAY 4:

I want you to identify one coping skill you currently use as a response to stress and anxiety. Ask yourself, "Is this coping mechanism helping me or hurting me?" Be honest with yourself and try to identify habits and behaviors that are either contributing to, or taking away from your happiness.

Now, ask yourself if there's something more productive you could do when stress presents itself in your life? Might it be appropriate to replace some of your current coping response with dancing? Personally, I have done this and it has made an enormous difference with my levels of stress and anxiety. Perhaps it could work for you too.

Now, I understand that everyone's situation is different. I'm not suggesting that dancing is the cure-all for stress and anxiety. You may need to talk to a professional to help you cope with the things in your life. However, I am saying that dancing can invigorate your body and mind and can help you feel better. While you can't avoid stressful days, you might be able to dance your way through a few of them!

List the things in your life that are causing your stress levels to rise and giving you anxiety.

_____

_____

_____

_____

_____

_____

_____

_____

_____

_____

_____

How do you currently respond to the stress and anxiety in your life? What are your "go-to" coping mechanisms? Are these good are bad?

_____

_____

_____

_____

_____

_____

_____

_____

_____

What are some positive ways to cope with the stress and anxiety in your life? (HINT: Dance more!)

_____

_____

_____

_____

_____

_____

_____

_____

_____

_____

_____

_____

_____

_____

_____

_____

Day 5 - Be Nice to Yourself

As a fitness trainer, I used to tell my students and clients, "NO PAIN, NO GAIN." It's not that I was trying to hurt people, it's just at the time I wholeheartedly believed that in order to get healthy, I needed to punish my body until it hurt. I was convinced that this was universally true for everyone.

Perhaps you've heard the "no pain, no gain" line too. Well, I now believe this is total nonsense. The fact is, pain is your body's way of communicating that something isn't right. Struggling through your workouts is the fastest way to destroy your body and your health.

In today's Discover Your Groove workshop I want you to keep in mind that the "no pain, no gain" way of doing things is a big, fat lie. But more than that, I want you to think about fitness in a different way.

Fitness and moving your body should never be a punishment. Instead, it should be a celebration of all the ways you can move, express and challenge your body. As Groovers, you should move and dance not because you hate your body, but rather because you love it. No matter what stage of life you find yourself in, you can always Groove and feel good.

I don't want you to fall victim to the "no pain,

no gain" lie anymore. Now, I'm NOT suggesting that you shouldn't challenge yourself in your workouts. Just be nice to your body and listen to its cues.

In today's workout - which is a challenging one - I want you to pay particular attention to the sensations you feel in your body. As you push your body, you may start to feel your muscles burn. That's OK. It's your body telling you it's working and getting stronger.

However, if there's a moment that doesn't feel right, or you feel aches or pain in your muscles and joints, then stop. Change what you're doing, or let your body rest and start again when you feel better.

Above all, I want you to approach today's Groove session with the perspective that you're doing this because you love your body and you want to treat it as such.

Here's your link to today's workshop and groove...

www.bodygroove.com/day5

ASSIGNMENTS FOR DAY 5:
As you go about your day today, be thinking about how you can treat yourself from a reward perspective. The way you move, talk, eat, think, etc. Reinforce how

amazing you are and how you need to give yourself all of the love and appreciation that you deserve. Today is day about being nice to yourself.

What are some ways that you can be nice to yourself today? Pick one thing you'll do today to be nicer to yourself and pay attention to how that makes you feel.

_____

_____

_____

_____

_____

_____

_____

_____

_____

_____

_____

_____

_____

_____

_____

Day 6 - You Weren't Born to Hate Your Body

In the beginning of this book I opened up about my struggle with bulimia. In today's Discover Your Groove workshop, I'm actually going to dive a little deeper into this struggle with the hope that what I've learned might help you.

Even though my story isn't pretty, I know that many of you can relate. Perhaps not so much with bulimia, but other dysfunctional things you might do in an effort to be accepted by others and to more easily love yourself.

While your personal story might be very different than mine, there's one thing we have in common... Just like me, you were not born to hate your body! Let me say that again. YOU WERE NOT BORN TO HATE YOUR BODY!

Hating your body is something that you've learned from people you associate with, what you're exposed to on television and in magazines, and especially from social media.

Think about a little baby or a toddler. They don't look at their bodies with any kind of contempt or dissatisfaction. And nor should you. It's time to unlearn your destructive thoughts and behaviors about your body. And that's what we're going to tackle in today's workshop and Groove...

Today's link...

www.bodygroove.com/day6

ASSIGNMENT FOR DAY 6:
For your workshop exercise today, I want you to "retrace your steps" so to speak. I want you to think through your own personal history and see if you can identify some of the influences in your life that cause you to have negative thoughts about your body.

For example, my negative body issues were the result of a number of factors. Family influence, MTV, fashion magazines, and working in the fitness industry. All of these things were causing me to doubt my true self worth and make me think that I wasn't enough.

What have you been exposed to that's creating a negative association with your body?

Once you can recognize the source of these destructive thoughts, you'll be better equipped to accepting the truth. That you weren't born to hate your body. Instead, you were born to love your body and to love yourself.

What experiences have you been exposed to, or are currently dealing with, that are negatively influencing the way you see and love yourself?

_____

_____

_____

_____

_____

_____

_____

_____

_____

Is it possible to remove the negative influences from your life? If so, how will you do that?

_____

_____

_____

_____

_____

_____

_____

_____

_____

Day 7 - Be Your Own Best Friend

Welcome back. To begin today I want you to close your eyes and picture your best friend. Now, if this person was overweight, would that stop you from caring about them? Would you be like, "Oh sorry Susan, you're a little too big right now for me to be friends with you anymore."

What if this person had some wrinkles, wasn't in great shape, or dressed different from you? Would that make even the tiniest bit of difference in the way you think about them?

If you're really this person's friend, it wouldn't make any difference at all. You would still love being around them and would accept them for whatever "flaws" they had. And that's brings me to the point of today's challenge.

It's so often easier to have grace and compassion towards others (especially your best friends) than it is to be gracious and compassionate with yourself. For some reason, it's just easier to see the dignity of others than it is to see your own.

I guarantee that you will never evaluate your friendship with someone else based on if they have a perfect butt. It just won't happen. So why are you losing sleep over the size of yours?

It's time to stop judging yourself!

Today, I want you to treat yourself the way you would treat your very best friend. Talk to yourself the way you would talk to them. Embrace your own unique, beautiful qualities like you would embrace theirs. Are you up for it? I know you can do it.

Here's today's link...

www.bodygroove.com/day7

ASSIGNMENT FOR DAY 7:

Your challenge for today is to hold yourself to the same standards you hold your friends to. If you can be compassionate towards them, and accept them for who they are, I want you to do the same for yourself.

Pay attention to the way your talk to yourself, think about yourself, how you move your body, and how you react to situations. Spend your entire day in a way that shows respect and love for yourself.

Now, I know this can be difficult and that it will take practice, but you can do it. You must do it!!!

If you're struggling with loving and valuing yourself, then today's challenge is especially for you.

What physical traits to you have that you tend to beat yourself up over? Do these traits accurately reflect who you are as a person or warrant whether you deserve someone's affection?

_____

_____

_____

_____

_____

_____

_____

_____

_____

_____

What are some ways you can treat yourself with the utmost level of respect today? Be specific.

_____

_____

_____

_____

_____

_____

_____

_____

_____

_____

_____

_____

_____

_____

_____

Day 8 - Take a Break

Congratulations. You've finished your first week and you should be very proud of yourself. Now, before we move on to your next week, I want to make one thing crystal clear. Wherever you're at with the challenge, whether you've done every single day, missed a few, or are taking it slower, it's all PERFECT just the way it is!

You might want to spend a couple of days on a particular topic. It might be a week before you move on. That's totally fine. The point of the Discover Your

Groove challenge is to help you make small, incremental steps in the right direction. Don't think that if you miss a day or two, that you've blown it. Just pick up when you're ready.

Judging yourself and comparing yourself to "what could've been" will do you no good. In fact, it'll reverse or delay any progress you could be making. So wherever you're at, let's start today from there.

With that said, today I want you to take a break. Take a break from introspection. Take a break from writing in your journal. Take a break from thinking too much. And instead, focus on getting the recovery that your body might need.

To help you do that, today's Groove focuses on relaxation and stillness and is from my from Mindful Movement series. It's all about taking a break and recharging your batteries.

Here's today's link...

www.bodygroove.com/day8

Day 9 - Meditation Made Simple

Sitting still and paying attention to your body, your breath and your mind is one of the most important things you can do to stay healthy, yet it's often neglected. People think they're being "unproductive" if they do these types of activities. However, from my experience, when you actually take the time to slow down, the results and outcomes in your life can speed up.

After the "awakening" I had where I realized I had to do things differently, I focused on figuring out a path to true health and happiness. A big part of this journey involved meditating. Now, I had never meditated before in my life, but something inside of me was telling me - actually shouting at me - to stop and be still. To take a moment to clear my mind and think about where I wanted my life to go. So, that's what I did.

At first, I wasn't very good at meditating. I actually thought there was something wrong with me as I couldn't seem to concentrate for more than a few seconds before my mind wandered, and I'd forgotten what I was supposed to be thinking about in the first place. However, as I kept up with it, I eventually got better and better at being still and allowing myself the peace it needed to function optimally.

In today's workshop lesson, we'll talk about how you can get started with this life-giving practice. I'll give you my take on how to introduce meditation into your daily practices, and then of course we'll get our groove on. So let's dive in!

Here's today's link...

www.bodygroove.com/day9

ASSIGNMENT FOR DAY 9:
I want you to join me in my "Introduction to Meditation" video that you'll find with the link listed above. As you watch this with me today, my hope is that you'll think about the things in your life that you'd either like to re-write, or the future that you're going to create. Be mindful of how you're going to create your own peaceful inner world.

What events in your life would you like to re-write? How will doing this change your life? Will it help your relationships, the way you talk to yourself, the way you act around others?

Day 10 - Learning to Love Yourself

Have you ever struggled to love your body? Have you ever felt like you can't love yourself until you achieve some "ideal" size or shape? Or, have you ever felt unworthy of someone else's love or attention because of the way you perceive yourself? I have, and I'll bet you have too.

I'll also bet that you've heard the saying, "Just love yourself." Well, that's good advice, but it can be a lot easier said than done. In fact, it's hard to even understand. I've come to learn that many of the women I work with struggle to grasp what "loving yourself" even looks like.

Can you relate?

For the longest time. I had no idea what loving myself meant, let alone how to actually do it.

Right now, if "loving yourself" seems out of reach – like it did for me for so long - and more of a far-fetched concept reserved for those OTHER women, consider this: You can begin to love yourself by first liking yourself!

Here's how that can work...

To begin, I want you to think about all the things

that you like about yourself. Big, small, it doesn't matter! Everything you can think of! For example, you could include things like your smile, your love of animals, your ability to cook a great meal, the way you help others, your sense of fashion, your compassion, or your appreciation for nature.

Now, as you do this exercise... please, please, please be kind to yourself! Too often we're our own worst critic. We give everyone room to breathe and make mistakes, but then suffocate ourselves with an expectation of perfection. (Remember the best-friend experiment? Treat yourself like you would your best friend.) As you do this, give yourself permission to run wild. Maybe even think of filling up your bathroom mirror with all of the wonderful things you like about yourself! As you do this my hope is that you'll start to see yourself as the amazing person you truly are.

Here's today's link...

www.bodygroove.com/day10

ASSIGNMENT FOR DAY 10:
Today is about creating your "like list". Write down the things you like about yourself. There are only two rules:

1. Make your list as long as possible and include as much as you can...

2. Remember to be kind.

Afterwards, keep this list handy. I want you to be able to remind yourself of how amazing you are.

So, why do I want you to do this...?

After a while of taking these small steps and recognizing how much you like yourself, something magical happens. One day you're going to look in the mirror, or have a thought about yourself, and you're going to realize just how much you really do love yourself. Best of all, you'll really mean it.

What are the things you really like about yourself? Write down everything you can think of. I want you to fill up this entire page and the next one.

_____

_____

_____

_____

_____

_____

_____

_____

Day 11 - Changing Your Inner Dialogue

Taking responsibility for your life begins with controlling your inner-world. Your thoughts, feelings, emotions... the way you talk to yourself. That's because the narrative you create in your inner-world eventually becomes your reality in your outer-world.

With that said, will you do a thought experiment with me? I'd like to ask you to think about a few scenarios for a moment.

Are you ready?

What it would be like if it were impossible to have negative thoughts about yourself?

What if every time you danced, you felt like the greatest dancer in the world, no matter how you moved?

What if when you examined your life, you only noticed the ways you were making progress towards improvement?

What if when you looked in the mirror, you only saw yourself positively and were never able to find any faults?

I hope you're starting to understand the purpose of why I'm asking these questions. I'd like for you to imagine a life where your inner dialogue and the way you think about yourself was always positive

How amazing would that be?

How would your life change if that were the case?

Do you think that without any negative thoughts weighing you down, you would feel lighter?

Would you be a happier person to everyone in your life, a source of encouragement to everyone you meet?

When you change your thoughts, ONE THOUGHT AT A TIME, your life changes too. You'll feel more confident, more in charge, more attractive. You'll be happier, emotionally healthier, and better able to be present with those around you. In short, everything will change for the better.

But, like so many things, it so much easier said that done. This workshop is designed to help you do it.

Here's today's link...

www.bodygroove.com/day11

ASSIGNMENT FOR DAY 11:

For your challenge today, I want you to write down some of the negative thoughts or self-talk that discourages you. Once you've identified some of these negative thoughts, I want you to ask yourself this question: who would you be if it was impossible for you to think those thoughts?

I appreciate that this his may take some time to really think about but it's so important. Even if you can't finish it all at once.

Also, remember that you are awesome!!

What negative thoughts or self-talk do you struggle with? What are the ways you get discouraged?

_____

_____

_____

_____

_____

_____

_____

_____

_____

_____

_____

_____

_____

_____

_____

_____

_____

What would you do, or how would your life change, if it was impossible to have these negative thoughts about yourself?

_____

_____

_____

_____

_____

_____

_____

_____

_____

_____

_____

_____

_____

Day 12 - Permission to Feel Amazing

Sometimes, you may not think that you're worthy or deserving of good things. That's because you've been to conditioned to believe a number of harmful lies. Things like, if you don't have a perfect body than you're not worthy of love. Or, that you're simply not allowed to feel amazing. Nothing could be further from the truth.

You are worthy right now of all the happiness you desire. You are allowed to feel amazing - right now. Today, we're going to take steps to help you feel this way.

Now, before we get started today, I want you to do two things:

1. Make sure you are alone. You'll see why in a minute.
2. I want you to remember that when you move your body your way, you can't get it wrong.

Are you ready? Then let's dive in.

Today's groove is just dancing individually with me.

There is no other formal Groove I have, but you're certainly welcome to Groove on your own.

Here's today's link...

www.bodygroove.com/day12

ASSIGNMENT FOR DAY 12:
As you go about your day today, I want you to give yourself permission to feel amazing. That will mean something different to each of you. However, allow yourself today to just feel great. You can do it.

Write down some of things, activities, hobbies, passions, etc., that make you feel really amazing?

_____

_____

_____

_____

_____

_____

_____

_____

_____

How can you incorporate more of these things into your life.

_____

_____

_____

_____

_____

_____

_____

_____

_____

_____

_____

_____

_____

_____

_____

_____

_____

_____

Day 13 - A Letter of Love

To help you embrace the truth that you really are special, I'm going to ask you participate in a small assignment. I'd like for you to write yourself a love letter.

That's right... a love letter.

Now, I want you to write this letter in a way that you would want a lover to write to you. What do you want them to say to you? What things do you want them to see in you? What things do you want them to appreciate about you?

One of the reasons I want you to write this letter is that sometimes we don't see what's right in front of us. Writing down your thoughts can allow you to see things more clearly, and help you identify and appreciate your talents and abilities. Things that you may have forgotten or overlooked.

I remember when I wrote myself a love letter. It was like...

"My dearest, sweet, Misty. I love the way that you have learned to trust your intuition. It's so beautiful to watch you blossom and flower and be an amazing woman. I love to see you, and your smile and how it lights up a room when you walk in. I love your empathy towards others and your passion to help people who are struggling."

In your letter nothing is off limits. You can write about anything you want. In my letter I mentioned superficial things like, "Your hair is so beautiful. I love your taste in clothes and how it expresses who you are. I love your smile."

I even bought up a few sexual things that I won't go into here. The point is, it's your letter and you can say anything you want.

So, what will you write?

Is it that you have a big heart? You're full of love, or that you're a really compassionate person. You're a great listener, a great friend and a great lover. Whatever it is, don't hold back because it's these things that make you unique, different, and special.

Will you accept this challenge? To write yourself a love letter and solidify what qualities you want the world to recognize about you. How you want to be seen. The things you wish others knew about you.

I know it can be difficult. But really give it a try because it will help you come to truly appreciate the things that make you amazing.

Today's workshop...

www.bodygroove.com/day13

Please note that in today's workshop you're going to need a simple handheld mirror. Or, you'll need to be in front of a mirror. You'll know why soon.

ASSIGNMENT FOR DAY 13:

I want you to write a love letter to yourself. Do it in such a way that you would want a lover to write it to you. Include things that you would want them to appreciate about you. You might include some of things you wrote down from day 10. Express all the things that you'd want in this letter and remember to have fun with it.

Write a love letter to yourself.

_____

_____

_____

_____

_____

_____

_____

_____

_____

_____

_____

_____

_____

_____

_____

_____

_____

_____

_____

_____

_____

_____

_____

_____

_____

_____

_____

_____

_____

_____

_____

_____

_____

_____

Day 14 - Your Gift to the World

If you don't know already - or have perhaps forgotten, please allow me to remind you. You are an amazing person. You have so many gifts that make you special and help bring light to others. Now that you're a couple of weeks into this Discover Your Groove challenge I really hope that you're starting to appreciate yourself in a whole new way.

Sometimes, it's easy for you to overlook how your uniqueness can be a blessing. You're so conditioned to just follow what everyone else is doing, that you don't embrace the things that make you special. However, it's typically only when you follow your own path, that you can really shine.

In today's workshop we're going to continue our exploration on the things that make you special. To do that we're going to do a meditation together. Now, if you remember from day 9, meditation can be easy. You can't get it wrong and there's nothing to master.

Today's workshop...

www.bodygroove.com/day14

ASSIGNMENT FOR DAY 14:

First, I want you to watch today's workshop with me and do the meditation. Once you've watched you'll be ready to record your thoughts about your gifts. Now, from previous days you should have started working on your list of things that make you special, or the things that you like about yourself. Today's list should be an extension of the list that you've already started.

The reason we're doing this again is that appreciating all that you have to offer, doesn't happen in one day. Plus, my hope is that after grooving for a couple of weeks with me, you're more attune to who you really are. So, dive a little deeper today in identifying the things that make you amazing. Think about how you can develop these attributes and how they can potentially help others.

And remember! Because you are unique, you should be different.

So, let yourself be different.

Don't try to follow anyone else's patterns.

Don't try to follow anyone else's rules.

Don't try to follow anyone else's anything.

Follow your own intuitive self.

Explore the deepest desires of your heart and what you can offer.

What makes you special? What are your gifts?

_____

_____

_____

_____

_____

_____

_____

_____

_____

_____

How can you use your gifts more to have a better life or to help more people?

_____

_____

_____

_____

_____

_____

_____

_____

_____

_____

Day 15 - A Reminder that No One Cares

For years, I made a HUGE mistake. I was SURE that everyone was constantly looking at me. I was 100% CONVINCED that everyone around me was judging me. So much so, that I spent my whole life doing everything for other people's approval. The clothes I wore, the car I drove, the area I lived in, even my job.

Everything about my life was done to keep up a certain "acceptable" appearance. In fact, my whole sense of importance and self-worth was dependent on making sure others approved of my choices. It's crazy to think about it now but I experienced severe anxiety about the possibility of losing the approval of others.

Here's the problem when you live your life trying to always please others, and being afraid of what they might think. You tend to hold back on the very things that make you special and unique. It stifles your creativity and imagination, and it prevents you from achieving your potential. This is true in every area of your life. Your work, your relationships, your health and wellness, everything!

I don't want you to feel like you can't be yourself. That's why in today's Discover Your Groove workshop we're going to explore ways to help you realize that because no one really cares about what you look like, you're free to follow your passions and to do the things that you really want to do.

Are you with me? Then let's do it.

Today's workshop...

www.bodygroove.com/day15

My Challenge to You.
When you dance today, will you be extra conscious to dance your own way. Put your special twist on every move you do. And above all... HAVE FUN!

ASSIGNMENT FOR DAY 15:
In today's workshop we're going to explore the idea that no one really cares what you look like and why this Groove Truth is so important to embrace. It's easy to say that nobody cares what you look like, but it's a whole different thing to actually live that way. That's why the techniques we talk about in today's video are SO HELPFUL!

Once you've watched the workshop, I want you to think about the following questions...

In what ways are you letting the judgements of others dictate your actions?

_____

_____

_____

_____

_____

_____

_____

_____

_____

What's one way that you can practice the Truth that No One Cares?

_____

_____

_____

_____

_____

_____

_____

_____

Day 16 - Practice Being Yourself

When you stop worrying about what others think, that's when you can embrace your own uniqueness. And the dance floor is a place where you can really practice this. Then, slowly but surely, you'll start to notice how this extends from the dance floor to your everyday life. It's amazing to see women all over the world who have done this and experienced a new level of confidence and self-love.

You can do the same!

In today's workshop I'm going to challenge you to practice being yourself. We'll do a dance that only requires you to walk. Walking is super simple, right? Yes, but as you'll soon see that this "walking" is not as easy as it sounds. After the workshop, as you do some Grooving with me you can continue to practice being yourself.

Check it out now. And while you're doing it, be fun, and playful, goofy, and mostly importantly, BE YOURSELF.

www.bodygroove.com/day16

ASSIGNMENT FOR DAY 16:

After you've done today's "walking" workshop, I want you to write down your thoughts about how you can practice being more yourself. Now, it doesn't need to be anything big. It could be as simple as wearing something different than you normally would. Or, it could be trying something new that fits your true personality. No matter what, try to figure out the things that will help you discover your true self.

What areas of your life can you be more authentic and more yourself?

Day 17 - You are Not Broken

Advertisers can't sell you something unless they can convince you that you have a problem or that you're broken. Once they do this, you're more likely to buy their product. I know that's cynical, but sadly it's the way it works.

Just think about a typical weight loss ad that features a person who is in perfect shape. These ads are intentionally crafted to make you compare yourself to these models. This reinforces the idea that because you don't look like them, there must be something wrong with you, and therefore you need fixing. Your "fix" is by buying whatever product is being advertised. Do you really think these models used the product in these ads to achieve their looks? Of course they didn't.

I don't want you to fall for these lies anymore. If you're not "model-skinny" that doesn't mean you're broken. If you don't have six-pack abs, there's nothing wrong with you. If your booty doesn't look like a famous actress, you're not deficient. And that's exactly what we're going to talk about in today's workshop.

www.bodygroove.com/day17

ASSIGNMENT FOR DAY 17:

You are not broken and you don't need fixing. You don't have to be a certain size, or look a certain way to have the life you desire. Now, that doesn't mean you shouldn't adopt practices that make you happier and healthier. However, don't adopt these practices based on the flawed belief that you need fixing. Do them because they make you feel good.

Are you doing things in your life, like dieting or exercising, because you incorrectly feel like you're broken? How can you change the way you think about these things?

_____

_____

_____

_____

_____

_____

_____

_____

_____

_____

_____

Day 18 - You're Supposed to Feel Good

For the longest time I used to beat myself up with exercise. I punished myself, and my students, in order to look and feel better. When I got home at night after teaching these classes I would collapse onto my bed, barely able to move because of the pain I felt. However, twenty years later, I'm nearly 50, and I'm virtually pain free. What has been the difference?

It wasn't until I started to honor and love my body, that I was able to figure out the best way to move it. I realized that I didn't need to kill myself to feel good or to see results. In fact, when I started moving my body in a more gentle manner, that's when I lost the weight that I'd been carrying around for so many years.

In today's workshop I talk about how you're supposed to treat your body with love and kindness. And, when you do this it can help you not only feel amazing on the inside, but also it can help you look great on the outside too.

I really think you're going to love what I have to say and that it's something that women - and men - everywhere need to hear.

Today's workshop...

www.bodygroove.com/day18

ASSIGNMENT FOR DAY 18:
I want you to think about the areas in your life where you can be nicer to yourself. Exercise can be a great start, but what about other areas? Perhaps the way you talk to yourself, the expectations you have. What areas of your life could benefit from you slowing down?

Here are some examples for you to consider:

- I am going to speak nicer to myself today.
- I am going to forgive myself more easily.
- I am going to treat my body with love.

You get the point. Now it's your turn to analyze your own situation and figure out how you can be nicer to yourself.

How can you be nicer to yourself today? How can you treat yourself with more love and kindness?

_____

_____

_____

_____

_____

_____

_____

_____

_____

What areas of your life are making you stressed? Can you slow down in these areas? If you do slow down in there areas, how will that help your life?

_____

_____

_____

_____

_____

_____

_____

_____

Day 19 - Overcoming Fear Restricted Movement

Are you ready to push some boundaries? I'm talking where you really let loose and discover things about your body and yourself that haven't explored before. Well, today's workshop lesson – which is also your workout – is going to help you do this. I want to warn you though; you can only truly discover these things about yourself when you embrace the idea that Your Way is the Right Way.

As mentioned, sometimes we're afraid to move or dance because of what others might think. We can even feel this way when we're alone. You can't let fear restrict the way you move, or live your life, or anything else for that matter. Today will be a small step in overcoming this.

Today's workshop...

www.bodygroove.com/day19

ASSIGNMENT FOR DAY 19:
Your way is the right way and it's time to start applying

this to EVERY aspect of your life. Think about where you are struggling right now because you're trying to mimic someone else? It could be in the way you exercise, speak, dress, think, socialize, or any number of things you do every day. Personally, I've found that when I stopped copying other people, that not only did my creativity increase exponentially, but also I become much happier.

What ways is your happiness, and creativity being held back because you're not doing things your own way?

Day 20 - Practice, Practice, Practice

Over the past few weeks we've focused on the first three Groove Truths...

1. You are Unique
2. No One Cares What You Look Like
3. Your Way is the Right Way

Now, it's time to really put them into practice because embracing these Groove Truths can be your individual road map to finding true health and happiness. However, no one can do it for you. You've got to be the one to do it, and it will take effort. That's because these Groove Truths aren't perfected overnight.

It can sometimes take doing thing many times before you notice a difference. However, step by step, inch by inch, you can transform the way you look at things, the way you treat yourself, and the way you love yourself. So, don't give up. You can do this.

Today's Groove...

www.bodygroove.com/day20

ASSIGNMENT FOR DAY 20:

There is no workshop to watch today. However, I do want you to Groove with me. As you do, I want you to practice the first 3 Groove Truths when you dance. I want this to be sort of like a mid-term test to see where you're at with the Body Groove way of doing things. Let this be a check-in as to see where you're doing great, and what areas you need a little help.

What grade would you give yourself for how effectively you implemented the Groove Truths in the way you danced today... A, B, C, D? How did this make you feel? What ways can you improve?

Day 21 - Rescue Yourself

Fairy tales all seem to have the same underlying story: Sweet young girl gets caught up in some terrible situation, and a knight/prince/hero swoops in to rescue her. Now, even though these are just fairy tales, we often live our lives as if they weren't. We feel trapped in some prison of unhappiness, all the while waiting for our rescuer to burst through the door and save us.

In today's workshop, I have some good news and some bad news. The bad news: there is no rescuer. No one's coming to help you. In fact, no one CAN help you. But the good news: you don't need a rescuer. The only person who can actually take responsibility for giving you the life you want is you. And in today's workshop, I'll explain why that's such great news. Today's workshop and groove...

www.bodygroove.com/day21

ASSIGNMENT FOR DAY 21:
If you've been hoping and expecting OTHER PEOPLE to rescue you, it's time to change your plan and plot a new course forward. I want you to take the

responsibility of your happiness off of others, and put it where it belongs: on your strong, capable shoulders.

What areas of your life have you been expecting others to rescue you? How can you take responsibility for these areas yourself?

_____

_____

_____

_____

_____

_____

_____

_____

_____

_____

_____

_____

_____

_____

_____

_____

_____

Day 22 - Healthy Selfish

Who are the people in your life who need you the most? Your spouse or partner? Your children? Parents? Colleague? Friends? Believe it or not, all these people need you to be MORE SELFISH!

When you take the time to actually take great care of yourself - even when that feels "selfish" - the people who depend on you the most reap the benefit. A stronger, healthier YOU is better for everyone!

For example, one area you could think about applying this is in your diet. I want you to EAT more selfishly. When you neglect yourself, it's easy to just grab whatever food is available. But why not be just a little "selfish?" Take the time to shop for real food that actually makes you feel good. Search out ingredients that you LOVE and that love you back!

Does it feel selfish to spend $4 on a big package of blueberries when a drive-thru burger is half the price? Maybe. But I want you to push yourself into that "selfish" zone and see what happens.

Today is about figuring out what areas of your life you can be "healthy selfish." Remember, you're doing this to be the best version of yourself. And that's when you can be the best for those who need you.

A great way to be "healthy selfish" is by taking time each day to Groove. So, Let's Groove!

Today's workshop...

www.bodygroove.com/day22

ASSIGNMENT FOR DAY 22:
I want you to write down 10 things that make you happy or that bring you joy, or that just help you feel good. Now, it could be up to 20 or 30 I'm just asking for 10 because that's a great place to start. I want this list to be your road map to your own personal joy. And keep in mind that what makes one person happy is different from what makes another person happy... we're all unique. Once you make your list, I want you to fill your life making these things happen.

Take the time. Do it for yourself, because no one's going to do it for you. Don't expect someone to go for a walk in the park for you. Don't expect someone to exercise for you or eat healthy food for you. Don't expect someone to meditate and develop a peaceful inner world for you. It will never happen. Don't wait for it. You have to cultivate these things for yourself. Take the burden of your happiness off of others and put it squarely where it belongs... with you.

Write down 10 things that make you happy, or where you could be more "healthy-selfish."

1. _____
2. _____
3. _____
4. _____
5. _____
6. _____
7. _____
8. _____
9. _____
10. _____

How can you do more of these things?

_____

_____

_____

_____

_____

_____

_____

_____

_____

Day 23 - Your 100 Year Old Self

Have you ever imagined being able to go back to your younger self and give yourself some advice? I have. Many times.

I think about the person I used to be and want to go back to her and tell her that she doesn't have to abuse herself. That she's loved. That she's perfect just the way she is. I'd like to tell her about all the amazing things she'll accomplish and to inspire her with confidence and self-assurance. Most of all, I'd like to tell her that she is enough.

What would you tell your younger self?

Although we may wish for it, obviously we can't go back and tell our younger selves what's what. But we CAN tell our current selves so many important truths for our future. And that's the gist of today's workshop. This is a MUST WATCH session and will give you so much insight into your life and what you need right now.

Are you ready? I'm going to introduce you to someone who will open your eyes in an amazing way, and give you the kind of advice we've been talking about. Spending just a few minutes with this person could be the most valuable time you spend with someone and I'm really excited for you to meet them.

WATCH THIS NOW!

www.bodygroove.com/day23

ASSIGNMENT FOR DAY 23:
How did you like meeting this person? Did they give you some good advice? I'll bet they did. Now, it's time to write down the advice that this person gave you and how you're going to apply it in your life.

What was the most important piece of advice your 100 year old self gave you?

_____

_____

_____

_____

_____

_____

_____

_____

_____

How will you implement this advice into your life?

_____

_____

_____

_____

_____

_____

_____

_____

_____

_____

What are some other pieces of advice you received that you would like to implement into your life?

_____

_____

_____

_____

_____

_____

_____

_____

_____

Day 24 - Your Future

How was meeting your future self? Did you give yourself some amazing advice? I'll bet it was awesome.

Today, we have a very special Discover Your Groove Workshop session where you'll be able to implement this advice into your life. As we discuss in our session today, it's vitally important to feel what your future is like. The more that you can sense what it feels like to live the life you want, the more you'll find yourself naturally heading towards it.

When you take time to "rehearse" living in the midst of your most delicious life possible, you'll find that as you move towards that future, it feels familiar, like you're returning to a home you've always known.

This is going to be great so let's get to it.

Today's workshop...

www.bodygroove.com/day24

ASSIGNMENT FOR DAY 24:
How did it go? Do you love the way your future looks?

Now, it's time to write down what you've started to imprint on your mind.

What does your future hold? What are your relationships like, your health, your happiness? What's the biggest difference between your life now and you future?

_____

_____

_____

_____

_____

_____

_____

_____

_____

_____

_____

_____

_____

_____

_____

_____

_____

_____

Day 25 - What's Holding You Back

Imagine for a second you owned a really expensive sports car, like a Ferrari or a Lamborghini. What if when you drove this car you never took it out of first gear. That you kept your speed to less than 20-30 miles per hour? Wouldn't that be a waste of the car's potential, the things it could do?

Now that you've learned so much about creating a more delicious life for yourself, I don't want you to miss out on what you desire or deserve! The time you've put into this challenge is a significant investment. The truths you've uncovered about yourself are priceless. The insights you've written down in your journal are worth their weight in gold! But, if you don't ever "get out of first gear" you won't benefit from all of your hard work.

Today is about building and flexing your Groove Muscles. It's about practicing the Groove Truths to develop the best life you can imagine.

Here's today's "Get out of First Gear" workshop...

www.bodygroove.com/day25

ASSIGNMENT FOR DAY 25:

After you watch today's workshop video I hope you're totally inspired to dance, and that you understand why it's so important to dance. It's all about giving you the space to flex your Groove Muscles and then watching your life become better for it. I don't want anything to get in the way of you experiencing this.

So, I want you to take a moment to identify what obstacles may prevent you from applying the Groove Truths in your life. I want these to be crystal clear in your mind so that nothing gets in your way from having the beautiful, amazing, delicious life that you deserve.

What obstacles or challenges could side-track your efforts to be healthy and happy?

_____

_____

_____

_____

_____

_____

_____

_____

What can you do to eliminate or minimize these challenges?

Day 26 - Soaking Up the Truth

Over the past few weeks you've learned about the Groove Truths and I hope you're really starting to implement them into your life. Now, as you know by now, the first and perhaps easiest place to apply these Truths is when you dance. And that's what I want you to focus on today. I simply want you to dance with me.

As you're dancing today – and always - I want you to keep these Groove Truths in mind. Allow them to soak into your entire body. Feel them with every movement. Hear them resonate in the music as you move your body exactly the way that is right for you. All the while remembering...

- You can't get this wrong.
- You are unique.
- Nobody cares what you look like.
- You have permission to feel amazing.
- And your way is the right way!!!

Dance with me now. Here's the link...

www.bodygroove.com/day26

ASSIGNMENT FOR DAY 26:

I hope you loved dancing with me today and that it helped you feel special and amazing. I want you to realize how dancing can help you be happy. And I want you to record your thoughts about this. That way, anytime you need a little pick-me-up, you can come back to today's workshop and remind yourself just how good it feels to dance.

How did you feel today while dancing with me?

_____

_____

_____

_____

_____

_____

_____

_____

_____

_____

_____

_____

_____

_____

Day 27 - What if...?

I want you to finish this sentence, "What would your life look like if.....?"

Answering this question is what I want you to explore today. And here's the really cool part, you get to be as creative as you want with your answers. That's right. Because you were born to thrive, today you're going to get a beautiful taste of just how delicious your life can be.

Here's what you MUST DO though!

You must think and dream BIG. Use your beautiful imagination to see what your life will look like when you have implemented everything we've talked about in this workshop.

What would your life look like if you were completely fearless? What would you do differently?

What would your life look like if you did things your own way, living your life on your own terms, by your rules?

That life is out there waiting for you, but you have to take responsibility to get it. To live life on your terms. Here's the link to today's workshop...

www.bodygroove.com/day27

ASSIGNMENT FOR DAY 27:

Today was actually the last workshop video in the 30 day Discover Your Groove Challenge. Don't worry, there are still plenty of Grooves left to do. But now that you're getting to the end of your 30 days I hope you're that you're inspired and excited about your future.

You probably noticed how my words today were similar to Day 24, when we talked about your future. I don't think this message can ever be repeated enough. Defining your future is such an important part of making your goals a reality. You must think and plan as much as possible about what you want and how you're going to get it.

With that said, look back at your answers from Day 24 and think about why these things are so important to you. Why do you want - or need - your future to look like this? Often, knowing the why of something is the determination you need to accomplish your goals.

For example, I was desperate to overcome bulimia and to love myself. But it wasn't until I figured out why I needed to do this that I was able to succeed. I needed to live a life where I loved myself. Where I treated myself with kindness. Where I could be myself. Otherwise I was literally going to die. That's pretty motivating.

Why do you want the future that you described on Day 24? What's your why?

What is your motivation for wanting the future that you described on Day 24? What's going to keep you motivated on the days where you feel like giving up?

_____

_____

_____

_____

_____

_____

_____

_____

_____

_____

_____

_____

_____

_____

_____

_____

_____

_____

_____

_____

_____

Day 28 - Just Dance

Today, let's dance and have fun. That's all I want you to do. However, as you dance with me will you do one thing? Will you forget about all the other things that are going on in your life that might be weighing you down? I know it can be hard, but will you put those things aside for a few moments and just focus on dancing with me? Will you dance with me today for the joy of dancing?

Forget about things like... I need to drop more weight, or I need to hit my number of steps today. Instead, just dance. That's it.

The link below to today's workouts will give you 3 dance routines that you can pick from. These range from more gentle and moderate... all the way up to really high energy. You decide what workout you want to do today.

But whatever you do.... JUST DANCE!!

Here's the link to your 3 routines...

www.bodygroove.com/day28

Day 29 - Your Beginning

As you near the completion of your 30 day Discover Your Groove challenge my hope is that you don't look at this as the end of your journey. Rather, as the beginning.

You were born to be great and to have an amazing life, but as you know, you're the only one who can make your life amazing. No one can do it for you.

My hope is that after nearly 4 weeks of practicing moving your own way, not worrying about what others think, following your intuition, being nice yourself, and so many other things, that you've started to see just how amazing and delicious your life can be.

Now, while 30 days is a good start, there's so much more to look forward to. Today is a reminder about how good it feels to move and enjoy your body. I really think you're going to love today's workshop... which is actually a private dance with me. As you dance, I want you to really pay attention to how good it feels to just move your body your own way.

Join me!

www.bodygroove.com/day29

ASSIGNMENT FOR DAY 29:

Today I want you to reflect on the last 30 days. What is different about you now? What did you learn about yourself? How will you use what you've learned to make your life the best it can be? Spend time thinking today how you're going to take what you've learned during these 30 days and use it as a foundation for the rest of your life. You can do this!

What did you learn about yourself over these past 30 days? What will you do to keep what you've learned part of your future life?

Day 30 - You Are Enough

Congratulations, you've reached the final day of your 30-day Discover Your Groove Challenge! You've learned all about the Groove Truths and how to implement them. You've practiced them and I hope they've helped you realize just how amazing you are.

I want to thank you from the bottom of my heart for trusting me and being with me these last 30 days. I know there have been days where it's been hard and you might have wanted to give up. There have been aches and pain, and a few tears along the way, but also some tears of joy, too.

I hope that you've gained so much through this process and that you're going to move forward with a determination to do whatever it takes to experience true, vibrant health. Why?

Because you are worth it. You are enough. You are amazing.

In the final session today, I'll be leading you through some of my favorite dances.

Here's the link...

www.bodygroove.com/day30

Chapter 9

What Others are Saying...

"You dance the way that your body feels comfortable with. I got fed up with workouts that you have to mimic and learn moves. I've lost over 30 lbs since I started and am so happy using Body Groove! It's the best investment I've made for my health." - Dana G.

"Easy to do at your own pace and level. Misty makes it fun and easy to accept yourself". - Lisa B.

"This was hands down the most perfect workout I've ever done." - Maryanne M.

"I started out slow sitting in my chair, then more weight started coming off and then I started getting up dancing more than ever. I lost 130 pounds thanks to Misty and Body Groove." - Penny H.

"Love the program. Love Misty. The work outs are fun and inspiring! This is the first program that I have continued for more than 30 days in a row! I come home from work, put it in, I don't dread it, I just do it! Thank you!" - Toni S.

"Misty is so incredible, motivational, and inspirational, she's a true gem that we've all been looking for. Thank you Misty." - Kim K.

"This is the best exercise program I've found that doesn't feel like exercise! I can do my own interpretation of the moves and in fact Misty encourages it. You CANNOT do this wrong! It doesn't matter what fitness level or age you are, this program can be done!" - Debbie R.

"This is an awesome program. It's so fun & you don't think you are working out but you most certainly are." - Alice B.

"Being able let my body move the way it needs to instead of trying to follow the regimented "follow me" instructors is wonderful! I move all over the place just listening to guiding words and suggestions all the while smiling and sweating." - Charlene T.

"Love it! It's the first time I don't feel like an idiot because I can't keep up with the routine. Making it truly my own personal workout is awesome!" - Kim A.

Dancing with Body Grove and Misty's positive encouragement, I feel more creative, happy, more confident, I smile more, and my 5'0" body stands a little taller. It's fun and having arthritis and osteoporosis ~ it feels wonderful to move my body in this way. - Cadie B.

I love that with Body Groove you get a full body workout without it being a hard core workout that takes all your energy and effort just to mimic the moves of the instructor. You Groove your own way and make it unique. That is all YOU!!! - Luanne K.

I would urge anyone of any age to give this a try....hate exercise? You will love Body Groove. - Karen M.

That is the beauty of Body Groove, it is your own dance, do it as you please and you can't get it wrong! - Taunya B.

I fell in love with dance again and felt liberated in my body for the first time in years! - Tessa C.

Groove has added so much to my day I cannot even begin to thank Misty enough for caring enough for others to create this easy, fun and doable program! Thank you Misty from the bottom of my toes, tips of my fingers, and center of my soul! - Stacy P.

I move better, stand straighter, have a bounce in my step, have a hell of a lot more confidence and am losing a lot of inches! Even my husband complimented on my toned booty. And its all down to you! Thank you so much. - Deborah W.

I am going on 49 with Fibromyalgia and Chronic Fatigue. I also had surgery to repair a tear in my left hip. The ability to Groove the way I feel is amazing. I have indeed lost some weight but that is not the most important thing. Nothing makes me feel whole like dancing does. That's why Body Groove is the best program ever. - Mary C.

For more Body Groove reviews...

www.facebook.com/bodygroove/reviews
www.bodygroove.com/pages/reviews